Non-Vascular Interventional Radiology of the Abdomen

Non-Vascular Interventional Radiology of the Abdomen

Ronald S. Arellano, MD

Massachusetts General Hospital
Harvard Medical School
Boston, MA, USA

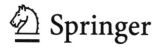 Springer

Ronald S. Arellano, MD
Department of Radiology
Massachusetts General Hospital
Harvard Medical School
Boston, MA, USA
rarellano@partners.org

ISBN 978-1-4419-7731-1   e-ISBN 978-1-4419-7732-8
DOI 10.1007/978-1-4419-7732-8
Springer New York Dordrecht London Heidelberg

Printed on acid-free paper

Springer is part of Springer Science+Business Media (www.springer.com)

This book is dedicated to my parents, Lola and Samuel Arellano, who made everything possible.

And to my wonderful and beautiful wife Hanna, who makes everything worthwhile.

Preface

The field of interventional radiology is a dynamic one, driven by the creativity and ingenuity of its practitioners. At its core, the field of interventional radiology is based on needles, guidewires, and catheters. With these tools, we can delve into the human body to diagnose and treat disease processes. In some case, we can even cure patients of their disease. I know of no other field in medicine that offers such satisfaction, excitement, and potential.

The purpose of this text is to provide basic principles and techniques of commonly performed nonvascular interventions of the abdomen. There are other more comprehensive texts that explore the latest and greatest that interventional radiology has to offer. This is not one of them. Instead, this book is intended to provide a foundation in the "when's, why's, and how's" of commonly performed nonvascular interventional radiology procedures of the abdomen. The chapters in this textbook are presented with this rationale in mind. Ultimately, the goal of this book is to be a handy and useful reference point for residents, fellows, and established radiologists who practice interventional radiology on a daily basis.

Ronald S. Arellano, MD
Boston, MA

Acknowledgments

I have been very fortunate to have trained at the University of California, San Diego and the Massachusetts General Hospital by some of the outstanding leaders in interventional radiology. Horacio D'Agostino, Thomas Kinney, Anne Roberts, Steven Dawson and Peter Mueller have all been incredible sources of inspiration for me. I am grateful for their patience and willingness to pass along their wealth of knowledge.

Contents

Preface.. vii

Acknowledgments.. ix

1 Patient Evaluation and Preparation.................... 1

Preprocedure Care.. 1

Review of Imaging Studies
and Medical History.. 2

Informed Consent... 3

Laboratory Evaluation... 4

Medications... 6

Insulin 6

Warfarin 6

Prophylactic Antibiotics.. 7

Procedural Care... 7

Conscious Sedation... 7

Postprocedure Care 10

Conclusion 11

References... 11

2 Image-Guided Percutaneous Biopsy 13

Indications.. 13

Contraindications 14

Equipment.. 14

Patient Preparation 15

Imaging Guidance 16

Ultrasound... 16

Computed Tomography... 17

Magnetic Resonance Imaging.............................. 17

Technique 18
    Fine Needle Aspirations...................................... 18
    Core Biopsy 18
Complications 19
Organ-Specific Biopsy.. 19
    Liver Biopsy... 19
    Spleen Biopsy 21
    Pancreas Biopsy 23
    Adrenal Gland Biopsy.. 24
    Renal Biopsy.. 25
Conclusion 27
References... 27

3 **Percutaneous Abscess Drainage** 33
Indications.. 34
Contraindictions... 35
Patient Preparation 35
Equipment 36
    Needles... 36
    Guidewires 36
    Directional Catheters 36
    Fascial Dilators 37
    Catheters 37
Imaging Guidance... 37
Drainage Technique 38
    Seldinger Technique... 38
    Tandem Trocar Technique.................................. 41
Drainage of Deep Pelvic Abscesses........................ 42
Solid Organ Drainage... 44
    Hepatic Abscess Drainage 44
    Splenic Abscess Drainage.................................. 46
    Renal Abscess Drainage 46
Complications 47
Postdrainage Management and Catheter Care 47
References... 49

4 Percutaneous Urinary Interventions 55
  Indications 55
  Contraindications 56
  Patient Preparation 57
  Patient Positioning and Imaging Guidance 58
  Anatomical Consideration and Selection
  of Puncture Site 59
  Access 60
    Ultrasound Guidance 60
    Fluoroscopy 61
    CT-Guidance 61
  Technique 61
    Percutaneous Nephrostomy
    for Nonobstructed Kidneys 64
    Nephroureteral Stent 66
    Technique 66
  Complications 67
  Follow-Up Care 67
  Suprapubic Cystostomy 68
    Technique 68
  References 69

**5 Percutaneous Gastrostomy
  and Gastrojejunostomy** 71
  Indications 71
  Contraindications 72
  Catheters 72
  Preprocedural Evaluation 73
  Technique 74
  Gastrojejunostomy 77
  Results 78
  Complications 78
  Follow-Up Care 79
  Conclusion 79
  References 79

6 Biliary Interventions 83
  Percutaneous Transhepatic Cholangiography 83
  Indications for Transhepatic Cholangiography 84
  Indications for Percutaneous Biliary Drainage 84
  Contraindications 85
    Imaging Guidance 85
  Technique 85
  Complications 89
  Percutaneous Management of Benign
  Biliary Strictures 89
  Management of Malignant Biliary Strictures 90
  Percutaneous Cholecystostomy 91
    Indications 91
    Technique 92
  Follow-Up 94
  Complications 96
  References 96

Index 103

1 Patient Evaluation and Preparation

Abstract The field of interventional radiology has evolved over the past 30 years into a well-established medical subspecialty. Increasingly, referring physicians rely on the imaging knowledge and technical expertise of the interventional radiologist to help guide and assist in patient management. As a result, it has become increasingly important for the interventional radiologist to have a fundamental knowledge about pharmacology, general anesthesia, and clinical management. This chapter presents essential elements that help establish a solid foundation for patient management and preparation for interventional radiological procedures.

Keywords Conscious Sedation • Laboratory evalution • Medical imaging

Preprocedure Care

All interventional radiological procedures begin with a consultation from a referring physician. With the exception of straightforward procedures, a discussion with the referring physician is always important. Challenging and complex cases always benefit from a discussion with the referring physician. This helps clearly establish the indications for the

R.S. Arellano, *Non-Vascular Interventional Radiology of the Abdomen*, DOI 10.1007/978-1-4419-7732-8_1,
© Springer Science+Business Media, LLC 2011

requested procedure, to delineate realistic expectations of the procedure, and to outline postprocedure care. This contact allows the interventional radiologist to discuss the pertinent imaging findings, and if appropriate, to offer alternative procedures or imaging tests before embarking on an invasive procedure [1]. It also allows the opportunity for the interventional radiologist to develop collegial working relationships with referring physicians [2].

Review of Imaging Studies and Medical History

A thorough review of all relevant imaging studies and medical history is an essential step in preparation for the procedure. Review of the pertinent medical imaging helps to establish the indications for the procedure and to make preliminary assessments regarding anatomy, patient positioning, and potential access routes.

The medical records should be reviewed to assess the overall medical status of the patient, to review current medications and to assess for potential contrast or medication allergies, and to determine the coagulation status of the patient. Particular attention should be given to comorbidities that render the patient unsuitable for having the procedure performed with the use of conscious sedation. The Physical Classification System of the American Society of Anesthesiologists (ASA) is a useful grading system designed to guide in selecting the appropriate type of anesthesia for surgery (Table 1.1). Consultation with an anesthesiologist is recommended for patients with limited head and neck motion and craniofacial abnormalities. Patients who classified as ASA class IV or V or uncooperative patients likely require general anesthesia for the procedure to be performed.

Table 1.1. American society of anesthesiology physical status classification.

Class	Patient health	Underlying disease	Limitations
ASA I	No systemic disease Normal healthy patient	None	None
ASA II	Mild systemic disease	Well-controlled	None
ASA III	Severe systemic disease	Controlled	Present but not incapaci- tated
ASA IV	Severe systemic disease that is a constant threat to life	Poorly controlled	
ASA V	Moribund patient who is not expected to survive without procedure		Incapacitated

Informed Consent

Written, informed consent is an integral component of any procedure. It is the responsibility of the physician who performs the procedure to get consent before the onset of the procedure. Informed consent must be obtained from the patient or their legal guardian in the case of minors or legally incompetent adults [3]. Informed consent allows the radiologist to explain the procedure to the patient and gives the patient or their representative the opportunity to address questions or specific concerns regarding the procedure [4, 5]. The discussion leading to informed consent should include the following:

- Indications and rationale for the procedure
- Risks and benefits of the procedure, including the consequences of refusing the treatment as well as alternatives

- Potential complications, including allergic reactions to contrast material or medication, and ways to manage them
- Possibility that the intended goals of the procedure may not be met

The signed written consent becomes part of the patients' permanent medical records.

Laboratory Evaluation

Several studies have demonstrated that indiscriminate preprocedural laboratory testing is neither useful, cost-effective, and contribute little to patient care [6, 7]. Therefore, coagulation testing should be tailored based on patient age, gender, and concomitant medical diseases [8]. When indicated, in most interventional procedures coagulation testing should include prothrombin time (PT), activated partial thromboplastin time (PTT), and platelet count [9]. Table 1.2 list commonly accepted thresholds for coagulation parameters. A typed and crossed sample of the patients' blood should be stored in the blood bank as preparation for managing potential bleeding complications.

Abnormally prolonged PT values should be corrected in the acute setting with transfusions of fresh frozen plasma (FFP). When possible, warfarinized patients should withhold their medication to allow normalization of the PT values. Depending on the clinical status of the patient, this may require temporary anticoagulation with intravenous heparin until the procedure is completed. The International Normalized Ratio (INR) is a commonly used test that measures the clotting time of blood. It is used to monitor patients taking warfarin and those with liver disease. It is generally accepted that an INR of approximately 1.5 or less is appropriate for most interventional procedures.

Table 1.2. Coagulation testing and factors that influence results.

Laboratory test	Normal range	Factors that affect results
Prothrombin Time (PT)	10–15 s	Cirrhosis
		Disseminated intravascular coagulation (DIC)
		Hepatitis
		Biliary obstruction
		Factor II, VII, X deficiencies
International normalized ratio (INR)	1.0–1.5	Same as for PT
Partial thromboplastin time (PTT)	25–35 s	Cirrhosis
		DIC
		Factor XII deficiency
		Hemophilias A and B
		Von Willebrand's disease
		Malabsorption
Bleeding time (BT)	1–9 min	Platelet aggregation defects
		Thrombocytopenia

The PTT also measures clotting time and is used to primarily monitor heparinized patients. Normal PTT values range from 60 to 70s. Prolonged PTT values are usually corrected by withholding heparin approximately 2 h before the procedure [10]. Patients with hemophilia or von Willebrand's disease may require transfusions of specific factors to correct abnormally elevated PTT values.

Platelets are an essential component of blood that aids in clot formation. Normal platelet values range from 150,000 to 400,00 per μl. Transfusions of platelets during the procedure is indicated for platelet counts <50,000 per μl and should be considered for platelet counts between 50,000 and 100,000 depending on the type of procedure and underlying medical condition of the patient. A variety of medical conditions and medications can affect platelet function.

Prolonged bleeding times should be treated with cryoprecipitate and/or desmopressin (DDAVP), and platelets.

Serum levels of blood urea nitrogen (BUN) and creatinine (Cr) should be checked if intravenous contrast is to be used for the procedure. Hemoglobin and hematocrit levels should be assessed and corrected whenever possible prior to the procedure.

Medications

Patients should take their regularly scheduled medications with a small sip of water on the day of their procedure. However, some exceptions apply.

Insulin

Insulin-dependent diabetics should consult with their endocrinologist or primary care physician for recommendations on how to manage their insulin on the day of their procedure. Patients taking Metformin (*Glucophage*) are at small risk of intravenous contrast material-induced renal failure. They should be advised to withhold their Metformin doses for 48 h before and after their procedure when intravenous iodinated contrast is necessary for the procedure.

Warfarin

Depending on the INR, warfarin should be held 5–7 days prior to the procedure, whenever possible, in order to allow correction of PT. It may be necessary in some circumstances to temporarily anticoagulate the patient with intravenous heparin while the patient remains off warfarin. Mildly elevated PT values at the time of the procedure can be treated with transfusions of FFP.

Prophylactic Antibiotics

Antibiotic prophylaxis is not indicated for all nonvascular interventional procedure, but should be applied to specific procedure types. Antibiotic prophylaxis is indicated for all biliary and genitourinary procedures [11]. Cephalosporins are most commonly used for gastrointestinal, genitourinary, and biliary procedures [12]. The combination of Ampicillin and gentamycin is also commonly used for genitourinary procedures.

Patients undergoing percutaneous abscess drainage usually have received preprocedure intravenous antibiotics. When this is not the case, broad-spectrum gram-negative coverage should be administered in the radiology suite. Antibiotic prophylaxis with Ampicillin and gentamycin is essential for patients with a history of bacterial endocarditis, cardiac valve dysfunction/anomalies or prosthetic heart valves who undergo biliary, urinary, gastrointestinal, or abscess drainages [12, 13].

Procedural Care

Conscious Sedation

The goals of conscious sedation are to provide relief of anxiety and pain and provide amnesia for the patient. These goals can often be met by the use of short acting anxiolytics and opioid analgesics. The ASA defines conscious sedation in a continuum of depths of sedation that range from mild sedation to general anesthesia (Table 1.3). With conscious sedation, patients have purposeful responses to verbal or tactile stimuli, have spontaneous ventilation and maintained cardiac function, and the airway need not be protected [14].

Patients undergoing conscious sedation should undergo physiologic measurements, such as heart rate, blood pressure, respiratory rate, and oxygen saturation at regular intervals (i.e., every 5 min). Additionally, the person providing the sedation should not be involved in other tasks. The person monitoring the patient should at no time be involved in the procedure, but should be focused solely on the comfort level and safe hemodynamic monitoring of the patient.

The combination of fentanyl and midazolam is most frequently used to provide conscious sedation for interventional procedures.

Midazolam (*Versed*) is a benzodiazepine that has anxiolytic as well as amnesic properties and a relative short half-life [15–17]. Dosing of midazolam is usually given in 0.5–1.0 mg increments until the desired level of moderate sedation is achieved. It can have respiratory depressant effects, especially when used in combination with other sedative, but has little cardiovascular effects. It undergoes hepatic metabolism. Its effects can be reversed by the benzodiazepine receptor antagonist Flumazenil [18].

Fentanyl (*Sublimaze*) is a synthetic opioid that is approximately 100 times more potent than morphine [19–22]. It has a 3–6 h half-life and is usually administered in doses of 25–50 µg until moderate sedation is achieved. Like other opiates, it has respiratory depressive qualities as well as cardiac depressive effects that can result in bradycardia. Fentanyl often causes nasal itching and can also cause nausea/vomiting and urinary retention. It undergoes hepatic

Table 1.3. Continuum of depth of sedation and anesthesia.

	Sedation		Deep	General anesthesia
	Minimal	Moderate		
Responsiveness	Normal response to verbal stimulation	Purposeful response to verbal/tactile stimulation	Purposeful response after painful stimulation	Unarousable
Airway	Unaffected	No intervention	Intervention may be necessary	Intervention likely required
Spontaneous ventilation	Unaffected	Adequate	May be inadequate	Frequently inadequate
Cardiovascular function	Unaffected	Usually maintained	Usually maintained	Can be impaired

Adapted from the American Society of Anesthesiology Practice Guidelines for Sedation and Analgesia by Non-Anesthesiologists. Anesthesiology, V 96, No 4, April 2002 metabolism. The opioid receptor antagonist Alexon reverses its effects [23].

Postprocedure Care

Hemodynamic monitoring should continue in the immediate postprocedure period. In- and outpatients should be transferred to their respective recovery areas only after a verbal report of the procedure and intraprocedural medications administered have been communicated to the receiving nurse. There should be a graduated decrease in observation intervals, such as every 15 min for the first hour, every 30 min for 2 h, then hourly for 2–4 h. Postprocedure monitoring should continue until the patient has regained baseline levels of consciousness and is hemodynamically stable [14]. Outpatients should be discharged with written instructions for postprocedure care as well as a telephone number with any questions that may arise. Table 1.4 lists ASA criteria for discharge.

Table 1.4. Discharge criteria after sedation and analgesia.

Patients should be alert and oriented; patients with initially abnormal baseline mental status should have returned to their baseline status.

Vital signs should be stable and within acceptable normal limits.

Outpatients should be discharged in the presence of a responsible adult who accompanies them home and is able to report any postprocedure complications

Outpatients and their escorts should be discharged with written instructions regarding postprocedure diet, medications, activities, and a phone number to call for any questions or in the case of an emergency.

Adapted from the American Society of Anesthesiology Practice Guidelines for Sedation and Analgesia by Non-Anesthesiologists. Anesthesiology, V 96, No 4, April 2002

Conclusion

This chapter has reviewed some of the essential points of patient preparation and evaluation that help establish a solid foundation for any procedure. The more familiar the radiologist is in all components of the procedure, the better he or she will be able to provide the highest level of patient care.

References

1. Becker GJ, Katzen BT. The vascular center: a model for multidisciplinary delivery of vascular care for the future. J Vasc Surg. 1996;23(5):907–12.
2. Katzen B, Kaplan J, Dake M. Developing an interventional radiology practice in a community hospital: the interventional radiologist as an equal partner in patient care. Radiology. 1989;170 (3 Pt 2):955–8.
3. Reuter S. An overview of informed consent for radiologists. AJR Am J Roentgenol. 1987;148(1):219–27.
4. Phatouros C, Blake M. How much now to tell? Patients' attitudes to an information sheet prior to angiography and angioplasty. Australas Radiol. 1995;39(2):135–9.
5. Mavroforou A, Giannoukas A, Mavrophoros D, Michalodimitrakis E. Physicians' liability in interventional radiology and endovascular therapy. Eur J Radiol. 2003;46(3):240–3.
6. Kaplan E, Sheiner L, Boeckmann A, Roizen M, Beal S, Cohen S, et al. The usefulness of preoperative laboratory screening. JAMA. 1985;253(24):3576–81.
7. Burk C, Miller L, Handler S, Cohen A. Preoperative history and coagulation screening in children undergoing tonsillectomy. Pediatrics. 1992;89:691–5.
8. Velanovich V. Preoperative laboratory screening based on age, gender, and concomitant medical diseases. Surgery. 1994;115: 56–61.
9. De Moerloose P. Laboratory evaluation of hemostasis before cardiac operations. Ann Thorac Surg. 1996;62(6):1921–5.
10. Horlocker T, Wedel D, Benzon H, Brown D, Enneking F, Heit J, et al. Regional anesthesia in the anticoagulated patient: defining

the risks (the second ASRA Consensus Conference on Neuraxial Anesthesia and Anticoagulation). Reg Anesth Pain Med. 2003;28(3):172–97.

11. Dravid V, Gupta A, Zegel H, Morales A, Rabinowitz B, Freiman D. Investigation of antibiotic prophylaxis usage for vascular and nonvascular interventional procedures. J Vasc Interv Radiol. 1998;9(3):401–6.

12. Spies J, Rosen R, Lebowitz A. Antibiotic prophylaxis in vascular and interventional radiology: a rational approach. Radiology. 1988;166(2):381–7.

13. De Gevigney G, Pop C, Delahaye J. The risk of infective endocarditis after cardiac surgical and interventional procedures. Eur Heart J. 1995;16:7–14.

14. Practice guidelines for sedation and analgesia by non-anesthesiologists. A report by the American Society of Anesthesiologists Task Force on Sedation and Analgesia by Non-Anesthesiologists. Anesthesiology. 1996;84(2):459–71.

15. Reves J, Fragen R, Vinik H, Greenblatt D. Midazolam: pharmacology and uses. Anesthesiology. 1985;62(3):310–24.

16. Davis P, Cook D. Clinical pharmacokinetics of the newer intravenous anaesthetic agents. Clin Pharmacokinet. 1986;11(1):18–35.

17. Garzone P, Kroboth P. Pharmacokinetics of the newer benzodiazepines. Clin Pharmacokinet. 1989;16(6):337–64.

18. Dunton A, Schwam E, Pitman V, Mcgrath J, Hendler J, Siegel J. Flumazenil: US clinical pharmacology studies. Eur J Anaesthesiol Suppl. 1988;2:81–95.

19. Zollner C, Schafer M. Opioids in anesthesia. Anaesthesist. 2008;57(7):729–40. quiz 741–2.

20. Trescot A, Datta S, Lee M, Hansen H. Opioid pharmacology. Pain Physician. 2008;11(2 Suppl):S133–53.

21. Inturrisi C. Clinical pharmacology of opioids for pain. Clin J Pain. 2002;18(4 Suppl):S3–13.

22. Peng P, Sandler A. A review of the use of fentanyl analgesia in the management of acute pain in adults. Anesthesiology. 1999;18(4 Suppl):576–99.

23. Goodrich P. Naloxone hydrochloride: a review. AANA J. 1990;58(1):14–6.

2 Image-Guided Percutaneous Biopsy

Abstract Image-guided percutaneous biopsy is a commonly performed interventional radiological procedure that plays an important role in patient care and management. It is a safe and effective procedure that is less invasive than surgical biopsy and can be performed using a variety of imaging modalities available to most radiologists. Increasingly, referring physicians rely on the expertise and skill of the interventional radiologist to obtain tissue specimens from organ systems within the abdomen and pelvis. Image-guided percutaneous biopsy is associated with low morbidity and mortality, and therefore it can be applied to patients who are too ill to undergo an operation. This chapter reviews the basic principles of image-guided percutaneous biopsy.

Keywords Fine needle aspiration • Core biopsy • Coaxial technique

Indications

The most common indications for image-guided percutaneous biopsy are to obtain tissue to [1] establish the presence of primary or metastatic malignant disease, [2] to assess for rejection in the setting of organ transplant, [3] obtain tissue in the setting of abnormal tissue function, (i.e., random

R.S. Arellano, *Non-Vascular Interventional Radiology of the Abdomen*, DOI 10.1007/978-1-4419-7732-8_2,
© Springer Science+Business Media, LLC 2011

liver biopsy for abnormal liver function tests) [4] to establish a benign diagnosis and [5] obtain tissue for culture for suspected infections [2, 3]. The decision to pursue image-guided percutaneous biopsy should be considered on an individual basis, taking into account the imaging and laboratory studies, overall medical condition as well as the potential risks of the procedure. Careful triage of biopsy requests helps to avoid unnecessary interventions.

Contraindications

Absolute contraindications include patients with uncorrectable coagulopathies or who lack a safe percutaneous trajectory to the targeted organ. Most bleeding disorders are correctable and are related to hepatic dysfunction, thrombocytopenia, or administration of anticoagulation medications. Commonly accepted coagulation parameters include an international normal ratio (INR) of 1.5 or less and platelets levels ≥50,000. Coagulopathies related to hepatic dysfunction or warfarin (Coumadin) can be reversed in the acute setting by transfusions of fresh frozen plasma, injections of vitamin K, or both. Similarly, transfusion of platelets at the time of biopsy is usually sufficient to correct thrombocytopenia. Other commonly used anticoagulants, such as aspirin and clopidogrel, should be held for at least 7 days prior to percutaneous biopsy whenever possible. Similarly, intravenous heparin should be held for approximately 2 h prior to biopsy.

Equipment

A variety of needle types are available for percutaneous biopsy [4, 5]. Most are classified into two general groups: aspirating and cutting needles [6, 7]. Aspiration needles are thinner gauge needles (typically 20–25-gauge) and are used to obtain material for cytological analysis. Because of their small gauge, these needles cause relatively little tissue disruption [8] and are associated with fewer bleeding complications. Cutting needles are larger, (typically 14–19-gauge) and are used to obtain material for histological evaluation [5, 9]. Various designs and cutting mechanisms for acquiring tissue specimens exist with these needle types [10]. All, however, serve the same goal of acquiring sufficient tissue for histological analysis.

Patient Preparation

Patient preparation begins with an assessment of the indications for percutaneous biopsy and review of the pertinent imaging studies. Review of the imaging studies also helps to plan the biopsy route and to consider options for patient positioning. The medical records, with attention to bleeding disorders or medications that may increase bleeding risk, should be carefully reviewed.

Most image-guided percutaneous biopsies can be performed with the use of intravenous conscious sedation. Occasionally, general anesthesia may be necessary, especially in pediatric or uncooperative patients. Patients should be advised to have nothing to eat or drink for at least 8 h before the procedure. Oral medications can be taken with a sip of water on the morning of the procedure. Diabetic patients should review their insulin requirements with the physician who manages their disease and make adjustments accordingly.

Unless the indications for biopsy are to assess for possible infection, intravenous antibiotics are not routinely administered. Written and informed consent should include a discussion of the potential risks and benefits of the procedure as well as a clear discussion regarding the indications for the procedure.

Imaging Guidance

Image-guided percutaneous biopsy can be performed with ultrasound, computed tomography (CT) and CT fluoroscopy. The choice of imaging guidance for percutaneous biopsy depends on a number of factors, but primarily relies on user preference and equipment availability.

Ultrasound

Ultrasound guidance is the preferred imaging modality for many interventionists [11–13]. Ultrasound guidance offers many benefits for image-guided biopsy. It is relatively low cost and allows real-time imaging without exposing the patient to ionizing radiation. Most biopsy needles are readily detectable by ultrasound and can be easily followed from the skin to the target organ. The relationships of the target and adjacent vasculature can be easily identified with ultrasound and thus aid in planning and guiding needle trajectory. Ultrasound also offers multiplanar imaging, further aiding in planning needle trajectory. The benefits of ultrasound, however, can be limited in patients of large body habitus in whom poor sound penetration results in poor image quality. Furthermore, lesions that are easily detected by contrast material enhanced CT or magnetic resonance imaging are not always readily detectable by ultrasound. Air from overlying or adjacent bowel or lung or lesions deep in the abdomen or pelvis may not be detected by ultrasound. High-frequency transducers (e.g., 7-MHz linear or phased-array) probes are usually sufficient for biopsy of superficial masses. Low-frequency probes, (e.g., 3.5 MHz sector probe) are necessary for deeper lesions. Ultrasound-guided biopsy can be performed using either freehand technique or with the use of an ultrasound needle guide.

Computed Tomography

CT is commonly used to perform a variety of percutaneous biopsies [7, 14–16]. CT guidance provides an alternative to US where poor image quality or identification of adjacent structures is not easily resolved. CT is especially helpful for biopsy of deep structures in large patients. While CT-guided biopsy lacks the multi-planar capabilities available with ultrasound guidance, gantry angulation can often create "windows" for safe access to the targeted structure [17]. CT fluoroscopy may allow more rapid imaging of the biopsy needle but image quality may suffer due to lower radiation dose used by this modality [18, 19]. The primary disadvantage of CT and CT fluoroscopy is that it exposes the patient and/or operator to ionizing.

Magnetic Resonance Imaging

Advances in equipment design have facilitated progress in magnetic resonance (MR)-guided interventions [20–22]. While not currently in widespread use, MR-guided biopsies have the following potential advantages [23]:

- MR offers exquisite soft tissue contrast and anatomic details. This allows the detection of lesion not readily available by other imaging modalities.
- The ability to elicit various pulse sequences can help define abnormal tissue that helps to specifically target tissue or areas within abnormal tissue.

- Multiplanar capabilities allow precise needle localization
- Provides imaging guidance without the use of ionizing radiation.

MR-guided percutaneous biopsies of the liver and prostate gland have been described [21, 24].

Technique

In general, the shortest and safest trajectory from the skin to the target lesion is preferred.

Fine Needle Aspirations

Fine needle aspirations are obtained by rapid reciprocating excursions of the needle tip within the lesion. Fine needle aspirations can be performed with or without gentle suction applied to the needle with a syringe. Greater suction is generated with larger needles. A sample of the specimen should then be smeared onto a glass slide and immediately placed into the appropriate fixative solution. Minimizing air exposure prevents air-drying and helps in the preservation of the specimen. Excess tissue samples can then be placed into a receptacle with appropriate fixative material. When lymphoma is a potential diagnosis, a dedicated fine needle aspiration should be designated for flow cytometry analysis. Similarly, tissue samples obtained for suspected infection should be processed to assess for Gram stain, culture, and sensitivities.

Core Biopsy

Cutting biopsy needles are designed to obtain small cylinders of tissue specimens for histological analysis.

The value of cutting needles is that they provide small cylinders of tissue that aid the pathologist in assessing tissue architecture.

Aspiration and cutting needles can be placed through coaxial introducers. This allows multiple samples, with either aspiration or cutting needles, to be obtained with a single puncture of the target organ.

Complications

Potential complications inherent to any biopsy include bleeding, infection, and unintended organ injury. The risk of neoplastic seeding is low [25–28]. The reported bleeding risk ranges from 0.1 to 10%, depending on needle size and target organ [2, 8]. Risks of infection and/or peritonitis are less than 5% [2]. Risk of pneumothorax is <1%.

Organ-Specific Biopsy

Liver Biopsy

Image-guided percutaneous liver biopsy can be divided into two general categories: random and focal and each type is performed to assess for different conditions. Random liver biopsies are performed using large gauge cutting needles in order to obtain a sample of hepatic parenchyma for histological analysis. Fine needle aspirations with a small gauge needle are seldom necessary. Random liver biopsies are usually performed in the setting of abnormal liver function tests, but other indications include assessment for rejection in the transplant patient or assessment for hepatic iron or copper deposition in suspected cases of hemochromatosis or Wilson's disease.

Most random liver biopsies can be quickly and safely performed with ultrasound guidance. CT can also be used, but exposes the patient to unnecessary radiation. The multiplanar capabilites of ultrasound allow percutaneous access to the liver via subxiphoid, subcostal, or intercostal approaches. When an intercostal approach is used, it is important to align the transducer within and parallel to the intercostal spaces. This minimizes acoustic shadowing from the ribs and improves image quality and needle visualization. Similarly, subxiphoid approaches should point away from the heart. Subcostal approaches must clearly identify gallbladder and bowel. Keep in mind that the position of the liver may change in the time interval between preliminary scanning and the actual biopsy. This is often due to changes in depth of respiration after the patient has been sedated. Smaller respiratory excursions in sedated patients often result in the liver assuming a higher position in the right upper quadrant, such that initial subcostal or subxiphoid trajectories are lost after the patient becomes sedated. When this occurs, an intercostal approach is obligatory.

Focal liver biopsies are aimed at obtaining tissue from specific hepatic masses for cytological and histological analysis (Fig. 2.1). Focal biopsies are necessary to assess for primary or metastatic liver disease and for possible infections. Biopsy with a coaxial needle is helpful for focal biopsies, as this requires a single puncture across the capsule and into the liver. Once the coaxial needle is in the desired location within the liver, removal of the inner styllette provides a conduit that allows multiple fine needle aspirations and core specimens to be obtained. The major complications associated with liver biopsy include bleeding, though pneumothorax, hemophilia, or tract seeding have also been described. When they occur, most bleeding complications occur at the time of the biopsy but may

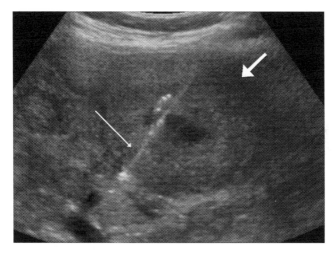

Figure 2.1. Ultrasound-guided biopsy of a focal liver lesion in the left hepatic lobe. The *thin white arrow* points to the needle. The *short white arrow* points to the liver lesion.

occasionally have a delayed manifestation. Most bleeding resolves with conservative management, but admission to the hospital and blood transfusions are occasionally necessary.

Spleen Biopsy

Splenic biopsy is indicated to assess malignant from benign lesions or to diagnose suspected infections (Fig. 2.2). Despite concerns of hemorrhagic complications image-guided percutaneous biopsy is a safe procedure. Tam et al. reported high sensitivity (83.4%) and diagnostic yield (92.3%) in a series of 156 patients who underwent image-guided percutaneous biopsy with 22-gauge needles [29]. Similar reports, including reports of core biopsy of the spleen, demonstrate high sensitivity and specificity with low complication rates [30–33]. In a series of 30 patients, Muraca reported

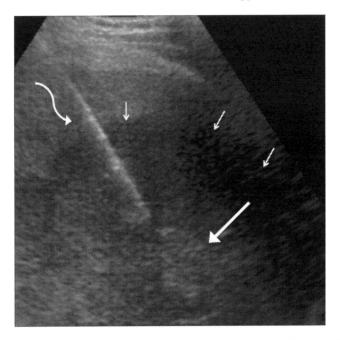

Figure 2.2. Ultrasound-guided biopsy of a splenic lesion. The *curved white arrow* points to the biopsy needle. The *long white arrow* points to an echogenic mass. The *short white arrows* outline the outer margin of the spleen.

no complications. Major complications, requiring emergency splenectomy are rare [33], and may have a higher association with tumor of highly vascular tumors [34].

Percutaneous spleen biopsies can be performed with ultrasound or CT guidance. When feasible, a coaxial needle is recommended as this reduces punctures of the splenic capsule, thus minimizing the risk of hemorrhagic complications. Traversing the least amount of parenchyma en route to the target lesion may help to minimize the bleeding risk [35]. A gelfoam suspension injected into the needle tract as the needle is withdrawn may help to minimize bleeding risk after splenic puncture [36].

Pancreas Biopsy

Because of the close anatomic relationship of the pancreas to the stomach and duodenum, most pancreatic masses are easily accessible for biopsy with endoscopic ultrasound (EUS). However, tissue sampling by this method is limited to fine needles aspirations. When tissue is needed for histological evaluation, percutaneous pancreatic biopsy can be performed. When core biopsies are performed, percutaneous biopsy of the pancreas is associated with high sensitivity and specificity for malignant tumors [19, 37].

The retroperitoneal location of the pancreas often lends itself to a direct posterior approach. When a posterior approach is not feasible, solid lesions can be biopsied via a transgastric route [38] (Fig. 2.3). The risk of pancreatitis may be increased when normal pancreatic tissue is included in the biopsy specimen [39].

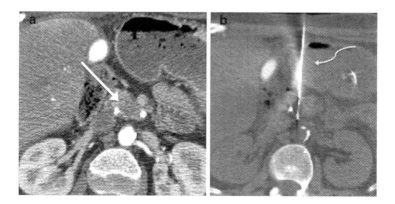

Figure 2.3. (a) Contrast material enhanced CT scan demonstrates a low attenuation lesion in the neck of the pancreas (*white arrow*). (b) *Curved white arrow* indicates the transgastric route of the biopsy needle in the pancreas neck mass.

Adrenal Gland Biopsy

Incidentally detected adrenal tumors are a common finding in abdominal ultrasound, CT or magnetic resonance imaging. Most incidentally detected adrenal tumors are benign adenomas that can be characterized using CT or MRI. Biopsy of the adrenal glands is usually performed to confirm metastatic disease or when CT or MRI cannot adequately characterize a benign adenoma [40, 41]. The sensitivity and specificity of adrenal gland biopsy are approximately 80 and 99%, respectively [42].

Percutaneous access to the adrenal gland can be achieved via posterior, anterior, or transhepatic approaches [43] (Fig. 2.4). Because of the high retroperitoneal location of the adrenal gland, a posterior approach with the patient in a prone position can be complicated by pneumothorax. This can be overcome by placing the patient in an ipsilateral lateral decubitus position. This displaces the lung out of the

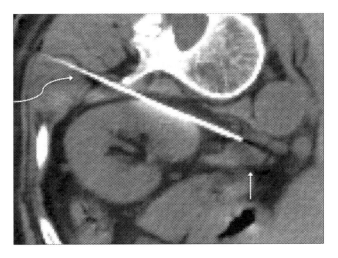

Figure 2.4. Computed tomography-guided percutaneous biopsy of a left adrenal tumor. The patient is in a lateral decubitus position. The curved white needle points to the biopsy needle and the short *straight white arrow* points to the left adrenal gland.

posterior costophrenic sulcus and often creates a safe trajectory to the adrenal gland that avoid lung altogether. When posterior or lateral decubitus positioning fail to displace lung, alternate approaches that go through lung, liver, kidney, pancreas, and spleen have been described [40, 44–47].

The possibility of a pheochromocytoma should be ruled out by biochemical testing for catecholamines or their metabolites [48, 49]. Failure to do so may result in severe hypertensive crisis [50].

Renal Biopsy

Percutaneous renal biopsy is performed for the evaluation of renal failure or to assess renal neoplasms [51–54] (Fig. 2.5).

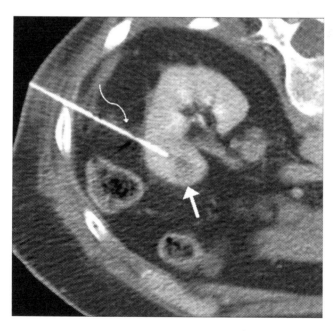

Figure 2.5. Computed tomography-guided percutaneous biopsy of a left renal cell carcinoma. The *curved white arrow* points to the biopsy needle. The *short white arrow* indicates the renal cell carcinoma. The patient is in a lateral decubitus position.

For appropriately triaged patients, percutaneous biopsy is a safe, reliable, and accurate method for assessing parenchymal disease and suspicious or indeterminate renal masses [54].

Nonfocal biopsy is typically performed in the setting of acute renal failure or to assess renal transplants in cases of suspected rejection [55]. Nonfocal renal biopsies are obtained using ultrasound guidance with a large-gauge cutting needle, typically 14- or 15-gauge (Fig. 2.6). With the patient in a prone position and using ultrasound

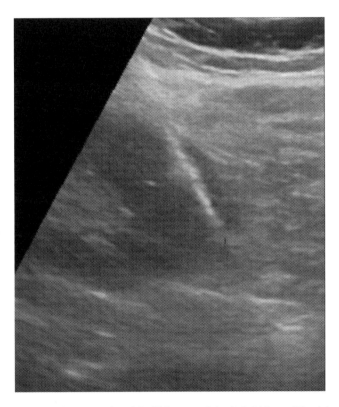

Figure 2.6. Ultrasound-guided biopsy of the left kidney. The biopsy needle should be directed toward either the upper or lower pole and away from the renal hilum so as to minimize the risk of renal hilar vascular injury.

guidance, the cutting needle should be directed toward either the upper or lower poles. It is important to obtain tissue from the renal cortex in order to maximize the yield of glomeruli in the specimen. Directing the biopsy needle away from the renal sinus helps to minimize potential bleeding complications.

Advances in tissue analysis and therapeutic options now available for the management of renal tumors have led to the value of image-guided percutaneous biopsy of focal renal masses. Published literature within the last decade demonstrates that percutaneous biopsy of renal tumors is safe. Serious complications are rare and a success rate of greater than 80% is attainable using percutaneous techniques [25, 56].

Conclusion

Image-guided percutaneous biopsy is a minimally invasive, yet valuable procedure that provides important and useful information for patient care and management. Most organs within the abdomen and pelvis are readily accessible using imaging guidance, and percutaneous biopsy should be considered the method of choice for establishing a benign or malignant process through tissue sampling.

References

1. Gupta S, Madoff D. Image-guided percutaneous needle biopsy in cancer diagnosis and staging. Tech Vasc Interv Radiol. 2007; 10(2):88–101.
2. Cardella J, Bakal C, Bertino R, Burke D, Drooz A, Haskal Z, et al. Quality improvement guidelines for image-guided percutaneous biopsy in adults. J Vasc Interv Radiol. 2003;14(9 Pt 2):S227–30.

3. Weigand K, Weigand K. Percutaneous liver biopsy: retrospective study over 15 years comparing 287 inpatients with 428 outpatients. J Gastroenterol Hepatol. 2009;24(5):792–9.
4. Betsill Jr WL, Hajdu SI. Percutaneous aspiration biopsy of lymph nodes. Am J Clin Pathol. 1980;73(4):471–9.
5. Gazelle GS, Haaga JR. Biopsy needle characteristics. Cardiovasc Intervent Radiol. 1991;14:13–6.
6. Haaga J, Lipuma J, Bryan P, Balsara V, Cohen A. Clinical comparison of small-and large-caliber cutting needles for biopsy. Radiology. 1983;146(3):665–7.
7. Chojniak R, Isberner R, Viana L, Yu L, Aita A, Soares F. Computed tomography guided needle biopsy: experience from 1, 300 procedures. Sao Paulo Med J. 2006;124(1):10–4.
8. Gazelle G, Haaga J, Rowland D. Effect of needle gauge, level of anticoagulation, and target organ on bleeding associated with aspiration biopsy. Work in progress Radiology. 1992;183(2): 509–13.
9. Nicholson M, Wheatley T, Doughman T, White S, Morgan J, Veitch P, et al. A prospective randomized trial of three different sizes of core-cutting needle for renal transplant biopsy. Kidney Int. 2000;58(1):390–5.
10. Gazelle G, Haaga J. Guided percutaneous biopsy of intraabdominal lesions. AJR Am J Roentgenol. 1989;153(5):929–35.
11. Otto R. Interventional ultrasound. Eur Radiol. 2002;12(2):283–7.
12. Johnson P, Nazarian L, Feld R, Needleman L, Lev-Toaff AS, Segal S, et al. Sonographically guided renal mass biopsy: indications and efficacy. J Ultrasound Med. 2001;20(7):749–53. quiz 755.
13. Liang P, Gao Y, Wang Y, Yu X, Yu D, Dong B. US-guided percutaneous needle biopsy of the spleen using 18-gauge versus 21-gauge needles. J Clin Ultrasound. 2007;35(9):477–82.
14. Aideyan O, Schmidt A, Trenkner S, Hakim N, Gruessner R, Walsh J. CT-guided percutaneous biopsy of pancreas transplants. Radiology. 1996;201(3):825–8.
15. Bernardino M, Walther M, Phillips V, Graham SJ, Sewell C, Gedgaudas-Mcclees K, et al. CT-guided adrenal biopsy: accuracy, safety, and indications. AJR Am J Roentgenol. 1985;144(1):67–9.
16. Lechevallier E, Andre M, Barriol D, Daniel L, Eghazarian C, De Fromont M, et al. Fine-needle percutaneous biopsy of renal masses with helical CT guidance. Radiology. 2000;216(2):506–10.

17. Hussain S. Gantry angulation in CT-guided percutaneous adrenal biopsy. AJR Am J Roentgenol. 1996;166(3):537–9.
18. Yamagami T, Iida S, Kato T, Tanaka O, Nishimura T. Combining fine-needle aspiration and core biopsy under CT fluoroscopy guidance: a better way to treat patients with lung nodules? AJR Am J Roentgenol. 2003;180(3):811–5.
19. Zech C, Helmberger T, Wichmann M, Holzknecht N, Diebold J, Reiser MF. Large core biopsy of the pancreas under CT fluoroscopy control: results and complications. J Comput Assist Tomogr. 2002;26(5):743–9.
20. Muller-Bierl BM, Martirosian P, Graf H, Boss A, Konig C, Pereira P, et al. Biopsy needle tips with markers–MR compatible needles for high-precision needle tip positioning. Med Phys. 2008;35(6):2273–8.
21. Tse ZT, Elhawary H, Rea M, Young I, Davis B, Lamperth M. A haptic unit designed for magnetic-resonance-guided biopsy. Proc Inst Mech Eng H. 2009;223(2):159–72.
22. Zangos S, Vetter T, Huebner F, Tuwari M, Mayer F, Eichler K, et al. MR-guided biopsies with a newly designed cordless coil in an open low-field system: initial findings. Eur Radiol. 2006;16(9):2044–50.
23. Weiss CR, Nour S, Lewin J. MR-guided biopsy: a review of current techniques and applications. J Magn Reson Imaging. 2008;27(2):311–25.
24. Stattaus J, Maderwald S, Forsting M, Barkhausen J, Ladd M. MR-guided core biopsy with MR fluoroscopy using a short, wide-bore 1.5-Tesla scanner: feasibility and initial results. J Magn Reson Imaging. 2008;27(5):1181–7.
25. Volpe A, Mattar K, Finelli A, Kachura J, Evans A, Geddie W, et al. Contemporary results of percutaneous biopsy of 100 small renal masses: a single center experience. J Urol. 2008;180(6): 2333–7.
26. Volpe A, Kachura J, Geddie W, Evans A, Gharajeh A, Saravanan A, et al. Techniques, safety and accuracy of sampling of renal tumors by fine needle aspiration and core biopsy. J Urol. 2007; 178(2):379–86.
27. Balzani A, Clerico R, Schwartz R, Panetta S, Panetta C, Skroza N, et al. Cutaneous implantation metastasis of cholangiocarcinoma after percutaneous transhepatic biliary drainage. Acta Dermatovenerol Croat. 2005;13(2):118–21.

28. Liu YW, Chen C, Chen Y, Wang C, Wang S, Lin CC. Needle tract implantation of hepatocellular carcinoma after fine needle biopsy. Dig Dis Sci. 2007;52(1):228–31.

29. Tam A, Krishnamurthy S, Pillsbury E, Ensor J, Gupta S, Murthy R, et al. Percutaneous image-guided splenic biopsy in the oncology patient: an audit of 156 consecutive cases. J Vasc Interv Radiol. 2008;19(1):80–7.

30. Lucey B, Boland G, Maher M, Hahn P, Gervais DA, Mueller PR. Percutaneous nonvascular splenic intervention: a 10-year review. AJR Am J Roentgenol. 2002;179(6):1591–6.

31. Muraca S, Chait P, Connolly B, Baskin K, Temple M. US-guided core biopsy of the spleen in children. Radiology. 2001;218(1): 200–6.

32. Keogan M, Freed K, Paulson EK, Nelson R, Dodd L. Imaging-guided percutaneous biopsy of focal splenic lesions: update on safety and effectiveness. AJR Am J Roentgenol. 1999;172(4):933–7.

33. Lindgren P, Hagberg H, Eriksson B, Glimelius B, Magnusson A, Sundstrom C. Excision biopsy of the spleen by ultrasonic guidance. Br J Radiol. 1985;58(693):853–7.

34. Hertzanu Y, Peiser J, Zirkin H. Massive bleeding after fine needle aspiration of liver angiosarcoma. Gastrointest Radiol. 1990;15(1):43–6.

35. Quinn S, Vansonnenberg E, Casola G, Wittich G, Neff C. Interventional radiology in the spleen. Radiology. 1986;161(2): 289–91.

36. Probst P, Rysavy J, Amplatz K. Improved safety of splenoportography by plugging of the needle tract. AJR Am J Roentgenol. 1978;131(3):445–9.

37. Itani K, Taylor T, Green L. Needle biopsy for suspicious lesions of the head of the pancreas: pitfalls and implications for therapy. J Gastrointest Surg. 1997;1(4):337–41.

38. Raczynski S, Teich N, Borte G, Wittenburg H, Mossner J, Caca K. Percutaneous transgastric irrigation drainage in combination with endoscopic necrosectomy in necrotizing pancreatitis (with videos). Gastrointest Endosc. 2006;64(3):420–4.

39. Mueller PR, Miketic L, Simeone J, Silverman S, Saini S, Wittenberg J, et al. Severe acute pancreatitis after percutaneous biopsy of the pancreas. AJR Am J Roentgenol. 1988;151(3): 493–4.

40. Liessi G, Sandini F, Spaliviero B, Sartori F, Sabbadin P, Barbazza R. CT-guided percutaneous biopsy of adrenal masses.

Experience of the technic in 54 neoplasm patients. Radiol Med. 1990;79(4):366–70.

41. Baker M, Spritzer C, Blinder R, Herfkens R, Leight G, Dunnick N. Benign adrenal lesions mimicking malignancy on MR imaging: report of two cases. Radiology. 1987;163(3): 669–71.

42. Welch T, Sheedy PN, Stephens D, Johnson CM, Swensen SJ. Percutaneous adrenal biopsy: review of a 10-year experience. Radiology. 1994;193(2):341–4.

43. Arellano R, Harisinghani M, Gervais D, Hahn P, Mueller P. Image-guided percutaneous biopsy of the adrenal gland: review of indications, technique, and complications. Curr Probl Diagn Radiol. 2003;32(1):3–10.

44. Krishnam M, Tomasian A, Davies L, Littler J, Curtis J. CT-guided percutaneous transpulmonary adrenal biopsy - a technical note. Br J Radiol. 2008;81(967):e191–3.

45. Price R, Bernardino M, Berkman W, Sones PJ, Torres W. Biopsy of the right adrenal gland by the transhepatic approach. Radiology. 1983;148(2):566.

46. Mody M, Kazerooni E, Korobkin M. Percutaneous CT-guided biopsy of adrenal masses: immediate and delayed complications. J Comput Assist Tomogr. 1995;19(3):434–9.

47. Kane N, Korobkin M, Francis IR, Quint L, Cascade P. Percutaneous biopsy of left adrenal masses: prevalence of pancreatitis after anterior approach. AJR Am J Roentgenol. 1991;157(4):777–80.

48. Shawar L, Svec F. Pheochromocytoma with elevated metanephrines as the only biochemical finding. J La State Med Soc. 1996; 148(12):535–8.

49. Singh R. Advances in metanephrine testing for the diagnosis of pheochromocytoma. Clin Lab Med. 2004;24(1):85–103.

50. Sood S, Balasubramanian SP, Harrison B. Percutaneous biopsy of adrenal and extra-adrenal retroperitoneal lesions: beware of catecholamine secreting tumours! Surgeon. 2007;5(5):279–81.

51. Burstein D, Schwartz M, Korbet S. Percutaneous renal biopsy with the use of real-time ultrasound. Am J Nephrol. 1991;11(3): 195–200.

52. Neuzillet Y, Lechevallier E, Andre M, Daniel L, Nahon O, Coulange C. Follow-up of renal oncocytoma diagnosed by percutaneous tumor biopsy. Urology. 2005;66(6):1181–5.

53. Volpe A, Jewett M. Current role, techniques and outcomes of percutaneous biopsy of renal tumors. Expert Rev Anticancer Ther. 2009;9(6):773–83.
54. Hara I, Miyake H, Hara S, Arakawa S, Hanioka K, Kamidono S. Role of percutaneous image-guided biopsy in the evaluation of renal masses. Urol Int. 2001;67(3):199–202.
55. Lefaucheur C, Nochy D, Bariety J. Renal biopsy: Procedures, contraindications, complications. Nephrol Ther. 2009;5(4): 331–9.
56. Lane B, Samplaski M, Herts B, Zhou M, Novick A, Campbell S. Renal mass biopsy–a renaissance? J Urol. 2008;179(1):20–7.

3 Percutaneous Abscess Drainage

Abstract Image-guided percutaneous abscess drainage (PAD) represents a major contribution by the field of interventional radiology to patient care [1]. Since the 1980s, it has evolved to become a well-established, minimally invasive procedure for the treatment of infected fluid collections in the abdomen and pelvis [2–6]. This chapter discusses the indications, techniques, and complications of PAD.

Keywords Subphrenic abscess • Seldinger technique • Tandem Trocar Technique • Pelvic abscess drainage

Introduction

Percutaneous abscess drainage involves image-guided percutaneous placement of a catheter to provide continuous drainage of an infected fluid collection [7]. This is in contrast to *aspiration,* defined as the evacuation of a fluid collection using either a needle or catheter, and then immediately removing the catheter or needle once the aspiration is completed [7]. Both are used to treat primary or postoperative infected fluid collections in virtually any organ system in

R.S. Arellano, *Non-Vascular Interventional Radiology of the Abdomen*, DOI 10.1007/978-1-4419-7732-8_3, © Springer Science+Business Media, LLC 2011

the abdomen or pelvis [8–10]. Because they are associated with reduced morbidity than surgical drainage, in many institutions they are the procedures of choice for treating abnormal fluid collections.

Indications

Specific indications for percutaneous abscess drainage (PAD) vary, depending on the imaging findings and clinical circumstances of the patient. In general, however, PAD is indicated when imaging studies reveal an abnormal fluid collection in a patient with clinical symptoms of pain, fever and/or leukocytosis. These clinical situations often arise in the setting of infectious or inflammatory conditions of the gastrointestinal or genitourinary systems, or develop following surgery [11–13]. Occasionally, imaging studies reveal

Table 3.1. PAD-1. Clinical conditions treatable by Percutaneous abscess drainage.

Complicated diverticular abscess
Crohn's abscess
Appendiceal abscess
Tuboovarian abscess
Postsurgical abscess
Gastrointestinal surgery
Pancreatectomy
Splenectomy
Hepatic surgery
Genitourinary surgery
Solid organ abscess
Hepatic abscess
Splenic abscess
Renal abscess

abnormal collections without clinical symptoms of infection. This is especially true of the elderly, severely ill or
immunocompromised patient. In such situations, needle
aspiration of the collection may be all that is necessary.
Table 3.1 lists conditions treatable by PAD.

When imaging studies confirm an abnormal collection and
the clinical setting of infection, PAD is indicated as long as a
safe percutaneous pathway exists and the patients' coagulation
status is within an acceptable range.

Contraindictions

Contraindications to PAD are relative, and include uncorrectable coagulopathy or unsafe percutaneous pathway to
the abscess.

Patient Preparation

Coagulopathies require correction prior to initiating the
procedure. Correctable bleeding disorders should be treated
in the acute setting with transfusions of fresh frozen plasma,
platelets or both depending on the abnormal coagulation
parameter. Most patients with suspected abscess have received intravenous antibiotics by the time the patient is referred
for drainage. If not, then broad-spectrum coverage should be
administered at the time of the procedure.

Most drainage can be safely performed with the use
of intravenous conscious sedation and local anesthesia.
Uncooperative patients, or those with severe medical
comorbidities (cardiac, pulmonary) or severe sepsis should
be treated with general anesthesia.

Equipment

The necessary equipment for PAD differ slightly depending on the technique (Seldinger or tandem trocar) and physician preferences. In general, most PADs require the following components: access needle, directional catheter, guidewire(s), fascial dilators, and drainage catheter.

Needles

Access needles range in size from 22- to 18-gauge. They can be biopsy type or sheathed needles of variable length. Prepackaged "single-stick" systems include a 22-gauge CHIBA needle, 0.018" guidewire and a three-component dilator system that allows conversion from 0.018" guidewire to either a 0.035" or 0.038" guidewire. Alternatively, 18-gauge sheathed needles accept either a 0.035" or 0.038" guidewire.

Guidewires

Guidewires are used to secure percutaneous access to collections. When Seldinger drainages are performed, the guidewire establishes percutaneous access to the collection and is necessary for deployment of the catheter into the collection. For purposes of PAD, 0.035" or 0.038" soft-tipped floppy or J-wires are used to establish access in the abscess. Thereafter, tract dilatation with the fascial dilators should be performed with a stiffer guidewire, such as Amplatz guidewire.

Directional Catheters

Directional catheters help negotiate guidewires within abscesses, especially those of irregular or complex morphology. They are also necessary for guidewire exchanges.

Fascial Dilators

Fascial dilators are necessary to expand the subcutaneous tissues and musculature before delivery of the drainage catheter. They should be tapered to fit over the guidewire. A floppy-tipped guidewire is often the initial guidewire used to establish access into an abscess. This is subsequently changed to a stiff guidewire to facilitate tract dilatation.

Catheters

Drainage catheters come in various sizes and configurations. In general, the catheter should contain multiple side-holes at the distal end to facilitate drainage, and an internal locking mechanism that helps to secure the catheter within the collection.

Imaging Guidance

Ultrasound, combined US/fluoroscopy or computed tomography (CT) is the imaging modality most frequently used to perform PAD [9, 14–17]. Lack of widespread availability of magnetic resonance imaging (MRI) scanners and MRI-compatible equipment limit the usefulness of this imaging modality for PAD [18], though this is likely to change in the future.

Ultrasound guidance offers of the benefits of multiplanar, real-time imaging without exposing the patient to ionizing radiation. This is of particular importance for pregnant or pediatric patients and in those patients with limited access to collections due to adjacent structures. Ultrasound guidance also allows the assessment of vascular structures that aids in planning needle and catheter trajectories. The combination of US/fluoroscopy is often helpful to gain access to collections that subsequently require fluoroscopic visualization of guidewire and catheter manipulations.

CT allows exquisite anatomic detail and clearly delineates the relationship of abscesses to adjacent vital organs [19]. Even though CT-guided PAD exposes the patient to ionizing radiation, the exposure is limited to a small volume of tissue, thus keeping radiation exposure to a minimum. Advances in CT fluoroscopy further limit the amount of radiation exposure to the patient [20].

Drainage Technique

Percutaneous drainages can be performed using either Seldinger or tandem trocar technique [6, 21, 22]. Familiarity with both methods is essential, as this allows the practicing interventional radiologist to have maximum flexibility in applying his/her expertise to a variety of clinical situations.

Seldinger Technique

PAD using Seldinger technique draws on the principles developed by Dr. Seldinger in the 1950s for safe access into the vascular system [23]. The elements of the Seldinger technique consist of four sequential steps: (1) percutaneous needle access into the collection; (2) guidewire placement into the collection via the access needle; (3) tract dilation; and (4) catheter delivery.

Initial percutaneous access into the collection is performed with the use of either ultrasound or CT guidance. The choice of needle size and type depends in most cases on operator preference; occasionally, it is dictated by the size of the percutaneous "window" to the collection. For most drainages, the initial needle is a 22-g or 18-g CHIBA needle, or 18-gauge sheathed needle. After the needle has been placed into the collection, 1–2 cc sample of fluid are aspirated and sent for microbiological and/or chemical analysis. The character and consistency of the fluid is analyzed to help determine catheter selection.

With the guiding needle in place, guidewire manipulations can begin. For "single-stick" systems, the 0.018" guidewire is advanced through the needle until so the stiff portion of the guidewire is within the collection. The needle is then withdrawn over the guidewire and replaced with the three-component stiffener/dilator/sheath apparatus. The stiffener/dilator components are then removed with or without the 0.018" guidewire and replaced with a 0.035" or 0.038" guidewire. When sheathed needles are used, the inner metal cannula is removed and replaced with either a 0.035" or 0.038" guidewire. Directable catheters may be necessary at this point to manipulate the guidewire into the desired position within the abscess, according to the size and shape of the collection. This type of manipulation is best accomplished with soft-tipped floppy or J-tipped 0.035" or 0.038" guidewire. This is particularly useful when draining subphrenic, (Fig. 3.1), deep pelvic or retroperitoneal collections that can develop along fascial planes. The soft-tipped catheter is then exchanged for a 0.035" or 0.038" stiff guidewire for fascial dilatation.

Fascial dilatation ideally should be performed with real-time fluoroscopic guidance. This helps to ensure that the guidewire does not kink and follows the course of the guidewire. Because this is not feasible with CT-guided drainages, the operator must rely on tactile sensation as the dilators are manipulated over the guidewire to ensure safe tract dilation. The subcutaneous tissues and

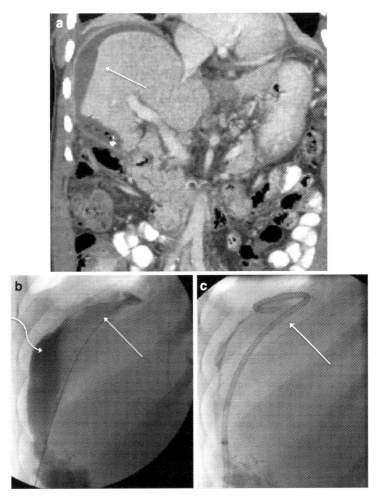

Figure 3.1. (a) Coronal CT scan of the abdomen that demonstrates right subphrenic collection (*white arrow*) that developed after partial hepatectomy. (b) Fluoroscopic image of same patient in Fig. 3.1a that demonstrates a guidewire (*straight white arrow*) that was placed into the right suphrenic (*curved white arrow*) collection using combined ultrasound/fluoroscopic guidance. Contrast material has been injected into the collection to define the margins of the collection. (c) Fluoroscopic image of same patient in Fig. 3.1b that demonstrates the final position of the drainage catheter (*straight white arrow*) that was placed within the collection.

musculature are serially dilated to the size of the drainage catheter. Occasionally, over dilatation by one French size is necessary in order to stretch fibrotic or scarred tissue.

With the percutaneous tissues adequately dilated, the drainage catheter can be easily advanced over the guidewire and into the abscess. With the catheter in position, the abscess is drained and the catheter is secured to the skin with a retention device. A three-way flow valve placed between the back end of the catheter and the drainage bag helps to facilitate catheter flushes.

Tandem Trocar Technique

Tandem trocar drainages can be performed with ultrasound and/or CT guidance [4, 24–26]. In contrast to Seldinger technique, tandem trocar drainage is a two-step process that consists of the following elements: (1) image-guided needle placement into the collection, and (2) trocar delivery of the drainage catheter alongside the guiding needle.

The initial image-guided placement of the guiding needle into the abscess is most commonly performed using ultrasound or CT guidance. For either type of imaging-guidance, the initial step requires placement of the needle from the skin to the abscess while avoiding critical structures. With ultrasound guidance, the needle is visualized real time as it passes from the skin to the collection. When CT guidance is used, the trajectory and distance from the skin the abscess are determined using electronic measuring tools on the CT workstation.

Once the needle is in place, a sample is withdrawn and sent for microbiological and/or chemical analysis. The consistency of the fluid is assessed and an appropriate size catheter is selected. A surgical blade is then used to pierce the skin, immediately adjacent to the guiding needle. With the drain-age catheter mounted onto the trocar needle/stiffener, the distance from the skin to the collection is marked on the catheter (a drop of blood from the skin puncture can be used). The catheter's tip is then placed on the skin at the puncture site and aligned perfectly parallel to the guiding needle. The catheter is advanced through the subcutaneous tissues and into the abscess all the while maintaining a trajectory parallel to the guiding needle. Once the appropriate distance is reached, the catheter is then released from the trocar needle/stiffener and advanced into the collection. Aspiration of pus indicates adequate placement. Repeat imaging should be performed to confirm position of the catheter tip within the abscess. The abscess should then be completely drained. A final set of images should be obtained after the abscess has been completely drained and the catheter secured to the skin.

Drainage of Deep Pelvic Abscesses

Access to deep pelvic fluid collections can be challenging due to the presence of a number of organs and bony structures in a confined space. Drainage of deep pelvic abscesses can be achieved via transabdominal, transgluteal, transvaginal, and transrectal routes using Seldinger or tandem trocar techniques [6, 25, 27–31]. The choice of approach often depends on operator experience, but in many cases the safest and shortest routes to the collection dictate approaches (Fig. 3.2). Transgluteal drainages provide access to collections high in the pelvis that are blocked from an anterior approach by overlying bowel, vessels, and bony pelvis. Access is via the greater sciatic foramen, often with the patient placed in a lateral decubitus or prone position. An angled gantry approach with the patient in the prone position

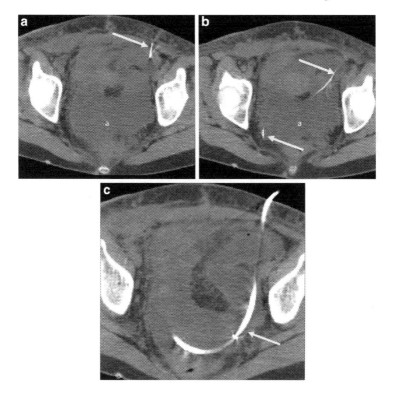

Figure 3.2. (**a**) Axial CT image of the pelvis that demonstrates the tip of a 20-gauge needle (*straight white arrow*) in the anterior aspect of a deep pelvic abscess (*a*). (**b**) Axial CT image of the pelvis that demonstrates 0.018″ guidewire (*straight white arrow*) that has been advanced into the deep pelvic abscess (*a*) through the 20-gauge needle. (**c**) Axial CT image of the pelvis that demonstrates the final position of a drainage catheter (*straight white arrow*) that has been advanced into the deep pelvic abscess.

may be necessary to find a suitable percutaneous window. Transgluteal entry into the pelvis should be as close as possible to the sacrum and below the piriformis muscle, whenever possible. This helps to avoid injury to branches of the internal iliac vessels and sciatic nerve [6].

Transrectal and transvaginal aspiration and drainages are commonly performed with ultrasound or combined ultrasound and fluoroscopically guided techniques [10, 25, 32–37]. These approaches are best suited for fluid collections in the inferior aspect of the pelvis, typically for abscesses in the prerectal space or cul-de-sac. An endoluminal probe, fitted with a needle guide, is used to localize and puncture the abscess. A guidewire is advanced using fluoroscopic guidance and a drainage catheter deployed over the guidewire after tract dilatation. Trocar drainages may require the use of a guiding sheath to direct the catheter into the abscess [26].

Solid Organ Drainage

Hepatic Abscess Drainage

Historically, hepatic abscess drainage has evolved from open surgical drainage combined with antibiotics to less invasive percutaneous drainage and antibiotic therapy [38]. Now, surgical debridement or hepatectomy is typically reserved for cases where percutaneous drainage fails [38–40]. Percutaneous hepatic abscess drainage is associated with high success rates (83–100%), good long-term outcome with low complication rates [41–43]. Pyogenic and amoebic liver abscesses are the two most commonly encountered hepatic abscesses [44], though fungal infections with *Candida species* can develop a complication of hepatic transplantations [45]. Pyogenic hepatic abscesses, often polymicrobial, are common in developed countries and have *Escherichia coli* and other enteric gram-negative rods as the major pathogens [46]. Staphylococcal liver abscesses, often associated with neutrophil disorders, are less common [47]. In the setting of infectious or inflammatory conditions of the gastrointestinal tract, the portal venous system acts as the conduit from the bowel to the hepatic parenchyma.

In developing countries, the trophozoite *entamoeba histolytica* is the most common etiologic agent of amoebic abscesses. Liver abscesses develop when amoeba breaches the gastrointestinal mucosal barrier and arrives in the liver via the portal vein. Abscesses consist of E. *histolytica* trophozoites surrounded by necrotic hepatic parenchyma and liquefactive cellular debris [48]. First-line therapy for amoebic abscesses is intravenous metronidazole [49] and percutaneous needle aspiration or percutaneous drainage is reserved for those who do not respond to therapy or who are at risk of rupture [50].

Hepatic abscess drainage can be performed with ultrasound or CT guidance, using Seldinger or tandem trocar technique, [41] (Fig. 3.3).

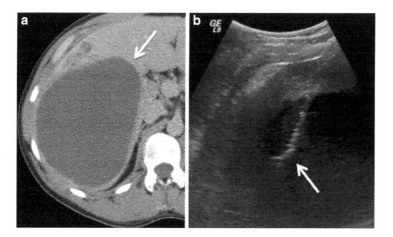

Figure 3.3. (**a**) Axial CT image of the liver that demonstrates a large hepatic abscess in the right hepatic lobe (*straight white arrow*). (**b**) Transverse axial ultrasound image of the liver that demonstrates a drainage catheter (*straight white arrow*) that was placed using trocar technique into the hepatic abscess.

Splenic Abscess Drainage

Splenic abscesses are an uncommon but potentially life-threatening clinical condition [51, 52]. Image-guided percutaneous aspiration and/or drainage of splenic abscesses have been demonstrated to a safe and effective organ-sparing alternative to surgery [53–56]. Most of the reported literature on splenic aspiration/biopsy describes ultrasound-guided techniques, though CT-guided drainages are also feasible.

Renal Abscess Drainage

Renal abscess drainage is an uncommon procedure. Percutaneous drainage provides immediate decompression as well as continuous drainage. When combined with antibiotic coverage, it is an effective nonsurgical alternative for the management of renal abscesses associated with high success rates [57–59]. Percutaneous drainage of renal

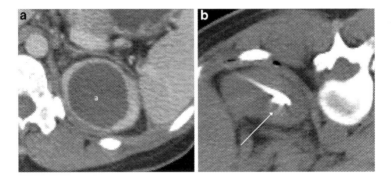

Figure 3.4. (a) Axial contrast material enhanced CT scan of the upper abdomen that demonstrates a left renal abscess (a). (b) Axial CT scan of the abdomen of the same patient in Fig. 3.4a that demonstrates drainage catheter in the left renal abscess (white arrow). The patient is in the prone position.

abscesses has outcomes similar to surgical debridement without the morbidity of surgical drainage [60, 61]. Ultrasound or CT guidance can be used, using either Seldinger or tandem trocar technique, (Fig. 3.4).

Complications

Major complications related to PAD are rare and range from 1 to 10% [7]. Major complications include septic shock, bacteremia that requires a significant new intervention, hemorrhage requiring transfusion and bowel transgression requiring a new procedure. Hemorrhage is more likely to occur in patients with uncorrected coagulopathies or when vascular structures have been traversed (Fig. 3.5). Additional major complications include superinfection of a previously sterile collection and pleural transgression that requires additional bowel or thoracic interventions.

Postdrainage Management and Catheter Care

Follow-up catheter care is an important component of the follow-up management of patients who undergo PAD. A three-way stopcock attached to the back-end of the catheter facilitates daily flushes to maintain patency. Catheters of any size can become occluded and therefore should be irrigated daily. Injection of 5–10 cc aliquots of normal saline into the catheter, followed by aspiration of fluid and reflushing of fluid, is usually sufficient to maintain catheter patency. Most catheters are secured at the skin using a plastic retention device and are allowed to drain into a collection bag. Recording of daily catheter outputs should

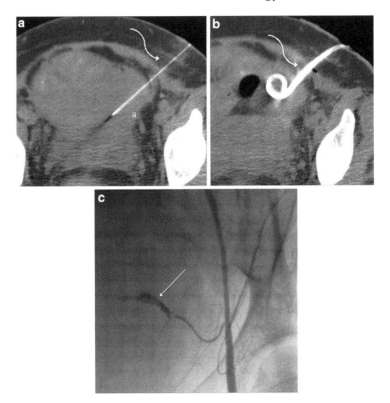

Figure 3.5. (**a**) Axial CT scan of the pelvis that demonstrates percutaneous placement of a 20-gauge needle (*curved white arrow*) into a deep pelvic abscess. (**b**) Axial CT scan of the pelvis of that demonstrates final position of the drainage catheter (*curved white arrow*) within the abscess. (**c**) Angiographic image of the left external iliac artery that demonstrates contrast extravasation of the inferior epigastric artery (*straight white arrow*). The patient developed acute pulsatile bleeding from the puncture site when the catheter was removed. The extravasation was controlled by coil embolization.

become part of the patients' daily medical record. If the patients' clinical condition fails to improve within 3–5 days after drainage, cross-sectional imaging studies may be necessary to assess the adequacy of drainage or for new collections. Additional drainages may be necessary for large collections or for abscesses that have become loculated after initial drainage. Intracavitary thrombolytics may facilitate catheter drainage, especially for complex collections [62–64].

Catheter removal should be considered when the following criteria have been met: improvement in the clinical status of the patient, improvement in laboratory tests, minimal catheter outputs (usually <10 cc/day), resolution of the abscess, and the absence of a fistula.

PAD of abdominal and pelvic collections plays an important role in the nonsurgical patient management. It is a safe and effective procedure and that represents a major contribution to medicine by the field of interventional radiology.

References

1. Ibele A, Heise C. Diverticular disease: update. Curr Treat Options Gastroenterol. 2007;10(3):248–56.
2. Al-Hilli Z, Prichard R, Roche-Nagle G, Deasy J, Mcnamara D. Iliopsoas abscess: a re-emerging clinical entity not to be forgotten. Ir Med J. 2009;102(2):58–60.
3. Eberhardt J, Kiran R, Lavery I. The impact of anastomotic leak and intra-abdominal abscess on cancer-related outcomes after resection for colorectal cancer: a case control study. Dis Colon Rectum. 2009;52(3):380–6.
4. Tasar M, Ugurel M, Kocaoglu M, Saglam M, Somuncu I. Computed tomography-guided percutaneous drainage of splenic abscesses. Clin Imaging. 2004;28(1):44–8.
5. Gerzof SG, Robbins A, Johnson W, Birkett D, Nabseth D. Percutaneous catheter drainage of abdominal abscesses: a five-year experience. N Engl J Med. 1981;305(12):653–7.
6. Zerem E, Hadzic A. Sonographically guided percutaneous catheter drainage versus needle aspiration in the management of pyogenic liver abscess. AJR Am J Roentgenol. 2007;189(3):W138–42.

7. Lee DH, Kim GC, Ryeom H, Kim JY, Kang D. Percutaneous paracoccygeal catheter drainage of deep pelvic abscesses using a combination of sonographic and fluoroscopic guidance. Abdom Imaging. 2008;33(5):611–4.

8. Carmody E, Thurston W, Yeung E, Ho CS. Transrectal drainage of deep pelvic collections under fluoroscopic guidance. Can Assoc Radiol J. 1993;44(6):429–33.

9. Buecker A, Neuerburg J, Adam G, Nolte-Ernsting CC, Hunter D, Glowinski A, et al. MR-guided percutaneous drainage of abdominal fluid collections in combination with X-ray fluoros-copy: initial clinical experience. Eur Radiol. 2001;11(4):670–4.

10. Lohela P. Ultrasound-guided drainages and sclerotherapy. Eur Radiol. 2002;12(2):288–95.

11. Soyer P, Fargeaudou Y, Boudiaf M, Hamzi L, Rymer R. Percutaneous abdominopelvic interventional procedures using real-time CT fluoroscopy guidance at 21 mAs: an analysis of 99 consecutive cases. J Radiol. 2008;89(5 Pt 1):565–70.

12. Harisinghani M, Gervais D, Hahn P, Cho CH, Jhaveri K, Varghese J, et al. CT-guided transgluteal drainage of deep pelvic abscesses: indications, technique, procedure-related complications, and clinical outcome. Radiographics. 2002;22(6):1353–67.

13. Akinci D, Akhan O, Ozmen M, Karabulut N, Ozkan O, Cil BE, et al. Percutaneous drainage of 300 intraperitoneal abscesses with long-term follow-up. Cardiovasc Intervent Radiol. 2005;28(6):744–50.

14. Ho KS, Hyup KS, Han H. Soo Kim S., Yeon Lee J., Hwan Jeon Y. Image-guided transvaginal drainage of pelvic abscesses and fluid collection using a modified Seldinger technique. Acta Radiol. 2008;49(6):718–23.

15. Seldinger S. Catheter replacement of the needle in percutaneous arteriography; a new technique. Acta radiol. 1953;39(5):368–76.

16. Gervais D, Brown S, Connolly S, Brec S, Harisinghani M, Mueller P. Percutaneous imaging-guided abdominal and pelvic abscess drainage in children. Radiographics. 2004;24(3): 737–54.

17. Rao S, Hogan M. Trocar transrectal abscess drainage in chil-dren: a modified technique. Pediatr Radiol. 2009;39(9):982–4.

18. Mcgahan J, Wu C. Sonographically guided transvaginal or tran-srectal pelvic abscess drainage using the trocar method with a new drainage guide attachment. AJR Am J Roentgenol. 2008;191(5):1540–4.

19. O'neill MJ, Rafferty E, Lee SI, Arellano R, Gervais D, Hahn P, et al. Transvaginal interventional procedures: aspiration, biopsy, and catheter drainage. Radiographics. 2001;21(3):657–72.
20. Butch RJ, Mueller P, Ferrucci JJ, Wittenberg J, Simeone J, White E, et al. Drainage of pelvic abscesses through the greater sciatic foramen. Radiology. 1986;158(2):487–91.
21. Gervais D, Hahn P, O'Neill M, Mueller P. CT-Guided transgluteal drainage of deep pelvic abscesses in children: selective use as an alternative to transrectal drainage. AJR Am J Roentgenol. 2000;175(5):1393–6.
22. Rose S, Kinney T, Roberts A, Valji K, Sanfeliz G, Miller F, et al. Endocavitary three-dimensional ultrasonographic assistance for transvaginal or transrectal drainage of pelvic fluid collections. J Vasc Interv Radiol. 2005;16(10):1333–40.
23. Sudakoff G, Lundeen S, Otterson M. Transrectal and transvaginal sonographic intervention of infected pelvic fluid collections: a complete approach. Ultrasound Q. 2005;21(3):175–85.
24. Men S, Akhan O, Koroglu M. Percutaneous drainage of abdominal abcess. Eur J Radiol. 2002;21(3):204–18.
25. Saokar A, Arellano R, Gervais D, Mueller P, Hahn P, Lee SI. Transvaginal drainage of pelvic fluid collections: results, expectations, and experience. AJR Am J Roentgenol. 2008;191(5):1352–8.
26. Maher MM, Gervais D, Kalra M, Lucey B, Sahani D, Arellano R, et al. The inaccessible or undrainable abscess: how to drain it. Radiographics. 2004;24(3):717–35.
27. Loren I, Lasson A, Lundagards J, Nilsson A, Nilsson P. Transrectal catheter drainage of deep abdominal and pelvic abscesses using combined ultrasonography and fluoroscopy. Eur J Surg. 2001;167(7):535–9.
28. Granberg S, Gjelland K, Ekerhovd E. The management of pelvic abscess. Best Pract Res Clin Obstet Gynaecol. 2009;23(5):667–78.
29. Nielsen M, Torp-Pedersen S. Sonographically guided transrectal or transvaginal one-step catheter placement in deep pelvic and perirectal abscesses. AJR Am J Roentgenol. 2004;183(4):1035–6.
30. Wroblicka J, Kuligowska E. One-step needle aspiration and lavage for the treatment of abdominal and pelvic abscesses. AJR Am J Roentgenol. 1998;170(5):1197–203.
31. Kuligowska E, Keller E, Ferrucci J. Treatment of pelvic abscesses: value of one-step sonographically guided transrectal needle aspiration and lavage. AJR Am J Roentgenol. 1995;164(1):201–6.

32. Petri A, Hohn J, Hodi Z, Wolfard A, Balogh A. Pyogenic liver abscess – 20 years' experience. Comparison of results of treatment in two periods. Langenbecks Arch Surg. 2002;387(1): 27–31.
33. Strong R, Fawcett J, Lynch S, Wall D. Hepatectomy for pyogenic liver abscess. HPB (Oxford). 2003;5(2):86–90.
34. Ng SS, Lee JF, Lai PB. Role and outcome of conventional surgery in the treatment of pyogenic liver abscess in the modern era of minimally invasive therapy. World J Gastroenterol. 2008;14(5):747–51.
35. Rajak CL, Gupta S, Jain S, Chawla Y, Gulati M, Suri S. Percutaneous treatment of liver abscesses: needle aspiration versus catheter drainage. AJR Am J Roentgenol. 1998;170(4): 1035–9.
36. Ferral H, Quiroz Y, Ferrari F, Hernandez-Ortiz J. Hepatic abscess: image-guided percutaneous drainage. Technique and indications. Rev Invest Clin. 1991;43(4):299–304.
37. Lee SH, Tomlinson C, Temple M, Amaral J, Connolly B. Imaging-guided percutaneous needle aspiration or catheter drainage of neonatal liver abscesses: 14-year experience. AJR Am J Roentgenol. 2008;190(3):616–22.
38. Kurland J, Brann O. Pyogenic and amebic liver abscesses. Curr Gastroenterol Rep. 2004;6:273–9.
39. Patterson J. Epidemiology of fungal infections in solid organ transplant patients. Transpl Infect Dis. 1999;1(4):229–36.
40. Yeh TS, Jan YY, Jeng L, Hwang T, Chao T, Chien R, et al. Pyogenic liver abscesses in patients with malignant disease: a report of 52 cases treated at a single institution. Arch Surg. 1998;133(3):242–5.
41. Mcdonald M. Pyogenic liver abscess: diagnosis, bacteriology and treatment. Eur J Clin Microbiol. 1984;3(6):506–9.
42. Stanley SJ. Amoebiasis Lancet. 2003;361:1025–34.
43. Chavez-Tapia NC, Hernandez-Calleros J, Tellez-Avila FI, Torre A, Uribe M. Image-guided percutaneous procedure plus metronidazole versus metronidazole alone for uncomplicated amoebic liver abscess. Cochrane Database Syst Rev. 2009;21(1):CD004886.
44. Goessling W, Chung R. Amebic Liver Abscess. Curr Treat Options Gastroenterol. 2002;5:443–9.
45. Alvi AR, Kulsoom S, Shamsi G. Splenic abscess: outcome and prognostic factors. J Coll Physicians Surg Pak. 2008;18(12): 740–3.

46. Tung CC, Chen F, Lo CJ. Splenic abscess: an easily overlooked disease? Am Surg. 2006;72(4):322–5.
47. Ferraioli G, Brunetti E, Gulizia R, Mariani G, Marone P, Filice C. Management of splenic abscess: report on 16 cases from a single center. Int J Infect Dis. 2008;13(4):524–30.
48. Zerem E, Bergsland J. Ultrasound guided percutaneous treatment for splenic abscesses: the significance in treatment of critically ill patients. World J Gastroenterol. 2006;12(45):7341–5.
49. Thanos L, Dailiana T, Papaioannou G, Nikita A, Koutrouvelis H, Kelekis D. Percutaneous CT-guided drainage of splenic abscess. AJR Am J Roentgenol. 2002;179(3):629–32.
50. Liu KY, Shyr Y, Su C, Wu C, Lee LY, Lui WY. Splenic abscess–a changing trend in treatment. S Afr J Surg. 2000;38(3):55–7.
51. Cronan J, Amis EJ, Dorfman G. Percutaneous drainage of renal abscesses. AJR Am J Roentgenol. 1984;142:351–4.
52. Gerzof S. Percutaneous drainage of renal and perinephric abscess. Urol Radiol. 1981;2(3):171–9.
53. Yen DH, Hu SC, Tsai J, Kao WF, Chern C, Wang L, et al. Renal abscess: early diagnosis and treatment. Am J Emerg Med. 1999;17(2):192–7.
54. Hung C, Liou J, Yan MY, Chang C. Immediate percutaneous drainage compared with surgical drainage of renal abscess. Int Urol Nephrol. 2007;39(1):51–5.
55. Shu T, Green J, Orihuela E. Renal and perirenal abscesses in patients with otherwise anatomically normal urinary tracts. J Urol. 2004;172(1):148–50.
56. Bakal C, Sacks D, Burke D, Cardella J, Chopra P, Dawson S, et al. Quality improvement guidelines for adult percutaneous abscess and fluid drainage. J Vasc Interv Radiol. 2003;14(9 Pt 2):S223–5.
57. Beland MD, Gervais D, Levis D, Hahn P, Arellano R, Mueller P. Complex abdominal and pelvic abscesses: efficacy of adjunctive tissue-type plasminogen activator for drainage. Radiology. 2008;247(2):567–73.
58. Haaga J, Nakamoto D. Computed Tomography-guided Drainage of Intra-abdominal Infections. Curr Infect Dis Rep. 2004;6(2):105–14.
59. Diamond I, Wales P, Connolly B, Gerstle T. Tissue plasminogen activator for the treatment of intraabdominal abscesses in a neonate. J Pediatr Surg. 2003;38(8):1234–6.

60. Mueller P, Vansonnenberg E. Interventional radiology in the chest and abdomen. N Engl J Med. 1990;322(19):1364–74.
61. Mueller P, Vansonnenberg E, Ferrucci JJ. Percutaneous drainage of 250 abdominal abscesses and fluid collections. Part II: current procedural concepts. Radiology. 1984;151(2):343–7.
62. Vansonnenberg E, Mueller P, Ferrucci JJ. Percutaneous drainage of 250 abdominal abscesses and fluid collections. Part I: results, failures, and complications. Radiology. 1984;151(2):337–41.
63. Oglevie S, Casola G, Vansonnenberg E, D'agostino H, Olaoide R, Fundell L. Percutaneous abscess drainage: current applications for critically ill patients. J Intensive Care Med. 1994;9(4): 191–206.
64. Wang I, Chen Y, Chen Y, Fang J, Hang C. Successful treatment of renal abscess with percutaneous needle aspiration in a diabetic patient with end stage renal disease undergoing hemodialysis. Ren Fail. 2003;25(4):653–7.

4 Percutaneous Urinary Interventions

Abstract Percutaneous nephrostomy (PCN) was first described in 1955 as a means to decompress a kidney obstructed. Since then refinements in technique and advances in equipment and image-guidance have established this procedure as an essential procedure for the interventional radiologist. While relief of hydronephrosis remains the leading indication for PCN today, access to the renal collection system serves other roles beyond the relief of hydronephrosis. This chapter reviews the indications, technique of PCN and nephroureteral stent placement; PCN is a mainstay of nonvascular interventions. Tract creation for stone extraction or other endoscopic manipulation is the same as that of PCN.

Keywords Hydronephrosis • Nephrostomy • Nephroureterostomy • Suprapubic cystostomy

Indications (Table 4.1)

The primary indication for percutaneous nephrostomy (PCN) is to temporarily alleviate urinary obstruction, most frequently as a result of urinary calculi. PCN is also used for

R.S. Arellano, *Non-Vascular Interventional Radiology of the Abdomen*, DOI 10.1007/978-1-4419-7732-8_4,
© Springer Science+Business Media, LLC 2011

Table 4.1. Indications for percutaneous nephrostomy.

Renal obstruction
Stones
Malignant urothelial tumors
Extrinsic compression of the ureters
Bladder tumors
Access for nephroureteral procedures
Percutaneous nephrolithotomy
Transrenal antegrade ureteral occlusion
Urinary diversion
Ureteral leaks
Urinary fistula
Hemorrhagic cystitis

urinary diversion to help heal urinary fistulas or leaks or hemorrhagic cystitis. PCN is also used as a precursor to more complex procedures, such as antegrade ureteral stents, percutaneous nephrolithotomy, or ureteral embolization. Less frequently, PCN is used to provide access for direct infusion of substances for stone dissolution, chemotherapy, and antibiotic or antifungal therapy [1, 2].

Contraindications

An uncorrectable coagulopathy or an uncooperative patient is the only real contraindication for PCN. Most bleeding disorders can be corrected with infusion of fresh frozen plasma or platelets. While no strict criteria exist to define acceptable levels of International Normalized Ration (INR) or platelets, commonly accepted parameters include an INR between 1.0 and 1.5 and platelet count ≥50,000 per cc. Patients with severe hyperkalemia (>7 mEq/l) should be treated with hemodialysis before undertaking the procedure.

Patient Preparation

Preparation for PCN begins with informed consent. In this process, the specifics of the procedure, including a discussion of the potential risks and benefits, are explained in detail to the patient. The postprocedure care of the catheter should also be explained to the patient. All relevant imaging studies should be reviewed with attention to regional anatomy, (i.e., location of the liver, colon, and spleen) and to determine the optimal approach to the kidney. The patient should be NPO for at least 6–8 h in order to safely carry out the procedure with the use of procedural sedation.

Periprocedural antibiotics, selected for the coverage of gram-negative anaerobes or specifically tailored to known urinalysis results, are given to help reduce the risk of sepsis [3, 4]. Intravenous administration is preferred because it provides rapid and reliable tissue levels and is less painful than intramuscular administration [5]. In the absence of clinical infection, antibiotic coverage with a first generation cephalosporin directed at gram-negative organisms can be used. When clinical infection is present and the results of the urinalysis are unknown, broad-spectrum coverage such as with ampicillin and gentamycin should be used [4].

Preprocedural laboratory tests, including a prothrombin time (PT), activated prothrombin time (aPTT), hematocrit level (Hct), and platelet count should be routinely ordered before the procedure. Correctable coagulopathies should be addressed prior to the procedure. Other tests, including serum blood urea nitrogen (BUN), creatinine, white blood count, and urinalysis should also be obtained prior to initiating the procedure.

Patient Positioning and Imaging Guidance

Patients are commonly positioned in a prone or ipsilateral prone oblique position. The prone oblique position helps to elevate the kidney. A foam pad placed under the patient may help to stabilize the kidney and to place the posterior calyces in a more vertical position. The ipsilateral upper extremity is flexed at 90° to facilitate positioning of the C-arm as close as possible to the patient [6].

Imaging guidance frequently involves ultrasound and fluoroscopy, though computed tomography can be used in unusual circumstances. Ultrasound guidance offers the benefits of real-time imaging and nonionizing radiation as the renal collecting system is punctured. Several access systems are available and all share the same basic components: needle, guidewire, and access sheath. Commonly used access systems include micropuncture sets that incorporate 22- or 20-gauge needles and a 0.018" guidewire. Larger sheathed 18-gauge needles with a trocar styllette can also be used and may be more readily visible with ultrasound guidance. Commonly used equipment for PCN is listed in Table 4.2.

Once the patient is properly positioned and the position of the kidney has been localized with ultrasound, the overlying skin is cleansed (Betadine or alcohol-based solution) and draped in a sterile manner. The patient is given appropriate medication for procedural sedation, (typically fentanyl or versed) and the puncture site is infiltrated with a local anesthetic, usually 1% lidocaine.

Table 4.2. Essential equipment for percutaneous nephrostomy.

Needles	22- or 20-gauge coaxial needle (CHIBA needle)
	18-gauge-sheathed coaxial needle
Guidewires	0.018" platinum-tipped guidewire
	0.038" floppy- or J-tipped guidewire
	0.038" stif f guidewire (Amplatz)
Dilator	6–14 French
Catheters	8–14 French catheter with locking pigtail
	mechanism

Anatomical Consideration and Selection of Puncture Site

A basic understanding of the renal anatomy is essential in order to safely obtain access into the renal collecting system. In particular, knowledge renal vascular anatomy can minimize bleeding related complications due to percutaneous access for nephrostomy and nephrolithotomy. At the level of the renal pelvis, the main renal artery divides into anterior and posterior divisions. Brodel's bloodless line is a relatively avascular plane of renal parenchyma between the anterior and posterior divisions of the renal artery and is an ideal entry point for access into the collecting system. The preferred site of entry into the renal collecting system is via a posterior calyx, through the papilla, ideally below the level of the 12th rib. This allows access through a point closest to the skin, and it is usually easier to pass a wire into the renal pelvis and down the ureter through a posterior calyx. Direct puncture of the renal pelvis or infundibulum should be avoided whenever possible due to the increased risks of vascular injury, potential for urinoma or catheter dislodgement.

Access

Ultrasound Guidance

Percutaneous access can be achieved using ultrasound or fluoroscopic guidance. Computed tomography is seldom used but can be employed in special situations in patients with anatomic anomalies [7]. Ultrasound offers the benefit of real-time imaging of the needle trajectory, visualization of adjacent structures and selection of a posterior calyx without the need for ionizing radiation [8] Fig. 4.1. Needle adjustments can be made in real time, thus potentially minimizing the

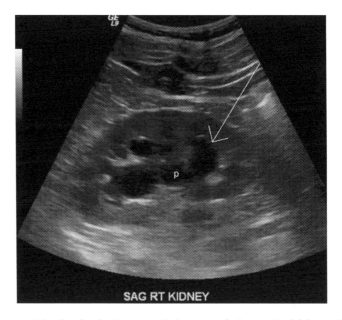

Figure 4.1. Sagittal ultrasound image of the right kidney that demonstrates a dilated renal pelvis (*p*), indicative of hydronephrosis. The *white arrow* indicates a dilated lower pole calyx selected for ultrasound-guided puncture as the initial step for percutaneous nephrostomy.

number of needle punctures into the kidney and because ultrasound does not use ionizing radiation, total radiation exposure time is kept to a minimum.

Fluoroscopy

Puncture sites for fluoroscopically guided PCN are ideally below the 12th rib to avoid transpleural and transpulmonary nephrostomy tracts – pneumothorax. When necessary puncture at the level of the 11th to 12th interspace is acceptable but a puncture site lateral to the paraspinal muscles is preferable to avoid transthoracic injury. When using fluoroscopy, the needle is aligned along the infundibulum, and the eye of the needle is directed into the calyx.

CT-Guidance

Computed tomography guided PCN is seldom used, except in unusual circumstances where altered retroperitoneal anatomy precludes ultrasound or fluoroscopically guided access [9].

Technique

The essential equipment necessary to perform PCN is listed in Table 4.2. After the collecting system is accessed with a suitable needle (Fig. 4.2), a sample of urine is withdrawn for microbiological analysis, including routine culture and sensitivity testing. Contrast material should be injected gently so as not to overdistend the collecting system. Overdistention should be avoided as this can increase the risk of bacterial seeding and the risk of bacteremia or sepsis. In general, contrast should be gently injected to

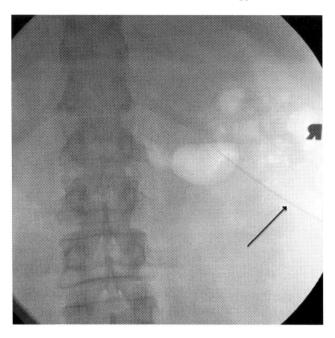

Figure 4.2. Fluoroscopic image of the same patient after ultrasound guided 20-gauge needle placement into the right kidney (*black arrow*).

identify the point of entry into the collecting system and renal pelvis. When no urine is readily obtained, a 10 cc contrast filled syringe can be attached to the needle via connecting tubing and slowly withdrawn, applying gentle negative pressure on the syringe. When urine is aspirated, the needle tip is likely within the collecting system, which can be confirmed with gentle injection of 5–10 cc of contrast (Fig. 4.3). Thereafter, a 0.018" platinum-tipped guidewire is gently advanced into the collecting system (Fig. 4.4). The guidewire should advance easily from the needle tip; any coiling or kinking of the guidewire is an indication that the needle tip is outside the collecting system. Once successful access

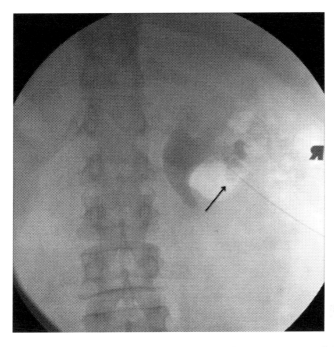

Figure 4.3. Antegrade nephrostogram that demonstrates satisfactory access into the dilated right renal collecting system via a lower pole calyx (*black arrow*).

into the renal collecting system is confirmed, wire exchanges are performed until a 0.038" guidewire is positioned within the renal pelvis or down the ureter. Thereafter, fascial dilators are used to widen the percutaneous tract. The nephrostomy catheter should be flushed and then mounted onto the stiffening cannula. Under fluoroscopic guidance, the catheter is then advanced over the guidewire until the tip just enters the renal calyx. At this point, the catheter is released from the stiffening cannula and advanced over the guidewire until the pigtail tip is positioned in the renal pelvis. The internal wire or locking device is then pulled to lock the pigtail catheter. Contrast injection is then performed to

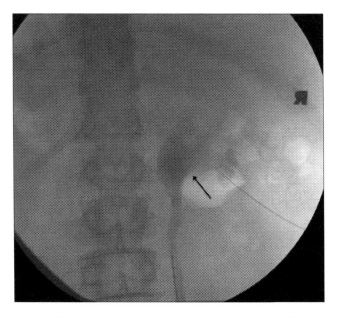

Figure 4.4. Fluoroscopic image that demonstrates a 0.018" guide-wire (*black arrow*) that has been passed through the 20-gauge needle and into the proximal right ureter.

confirm the final position of the catheter in the renal pelvis (Fig. 4.5). In most cases, an 8 Fr catheter is sufficient to decompress the kidney. If transrenal interventions of the collecting system are necessary, the catheter can be easily upsized under fluoroscopic guidance.

Percutaneous Nephrostomy for Nonobstructed Kidneys

Occasionally, PCN is necessary for nonobstructed kid-neys, (i.e., urinary diversion for urinary leaks, fistulas or with nondilated ureteral obstruction). In these situations, accessing the renal collecting system can pose unique

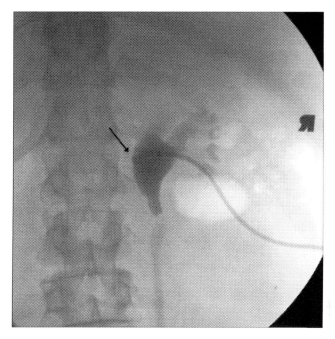

Figure 4.5. Fluoroscopic image that demonstrates final position of the percutaneous nephrostomy catheter (*black arrow*) into the right renal pelvis.

challenges due to poor visualization and nondilated collecting system. When PCN is indicated for urinary diversion in the setting of normal serum creatinine, iodinated contrast is administered intravenously and after approximately 5 min, a 22-gauge needle is directed into the renal pelvis using fluoroscopic guidance. Once aspiration of urine is confirmed, additional contrast is injected directly into the renal pelvis to opacify the calyces, or if possible, directly into a suitable calyx. When elevation of the serum creatinine precludes the use of intravenous contrast, carbon dioxide maybe considered as a contrast agent. The gas acts as a contrast and that rises within the collecting system to fill posterior, nondependent calyces. However, aspiration of urine must always be confirmed prior to injection of air in order to avoid intravascular injection of air and possible air embolism. Thereafter, iodinated contrast or 5–10 ml of carbon dioxide can be used to confirm needle position in the collecting system. Once a posterior calyx is identified, the overlying skin is anesthetized and punctured using an 18-gauge sheathed needle. When the calyx has been properly accessed, the needle is removed from the sheath and replaced with a 0.035" guidewire. When the guidewire has been successfully advanced into the renal pelvis or down the ureter, the sheath is advanced over the guidewire, which is then replaced with a 0.038" stiff guidewire and the remainder of the procedure is carried as for a dilated system [10].

Nephroureteral Stent

Nephroureteral stents provide access to renal collecting system in the same manner as nephrostomy catheters but allow for primary internal drainage. They are an alternative to double-J internal ureteral stents that are used to provide drainage across points of ureteral obstruction. These catheters extend the length from the skin to the urinary bladder and should be so positioned that the side holes extend proximal as well as distal to the point of obstruction.

Technique

Image-guided access to the renal collecting system is identical to that of PCN. A directional angiographic catheter combined with a soft-tip catheter is then used to negotiate the guidewire across the point of ureteral narrowing and into the urinary bladder. The soft-tip catheter is then exchanged for a stiff working wire. The nephroureteral stent is advanced over the stiff wire, with or without the use of a peel-away sheath, and into the urinary bladder. The catheter should be pushed off the metal stiff once the tip enters collecting system so as to avoid renal colic that can be induced by the metal stiffener as it is advanced deep into the collecting system. Catheters that are 22-cm in length accommodate most patients; however, longer catheters are also available if needed.

Complications

Major complications associated with PCN and nephroureteral stent placement are rare [11], and the risk can be kept low by proper patient selection and technique [12]. The most serious complication is renal hemorrhage and is often the result of pseudoaneurysm that can be treated by selective embolization [13]. Sepsis (0.3–4.7%) is not as frequently encountered when compared to biliary interventions, unless the patient suffers from gross pyuria [4].

Injury to adjacent structures is a potential problem that is easily overcome by careful review of cross-sections imaging studies, when available, [11, 13]. Colonic injuries are rare and when they occur seldom require surgical correction [14, 15]. Pleural complications are associated with upper pole accesses and may result in the development of pleural effusions or pneumothorax [16].

Follow-Up Care

Routine follow-up of hospitalized patients includes daily evaluation of urine output, diminution of hematuria, and gradual resolution of flank pain following PCN [17]. Patients who require long-term external drainage should undergo routine schedule catheter exchanges before they become occluded, usually from encrustation of the catheter tip and side hole by mucous, debris, or urinary salts.

Suprapubic Cystostomy

The first line of therapy for patients with chronic bladder or urethral outlet obstruction is urinary diversion by use of a Foley catheter. When this is not feasible due to high-grade obstruction, suprapubic cystostomy offers a safe and effective alternative to drainage. Suprapubic pubic cystostomy is also often requested for patients with neurogenic bladders who are unable to perform self-catheterizations.

Technique

Percutaneous suprapubic cystostomy can be safely performed with the use of ultrasound guidance or with combined ultrasound and fluoroscopic guidance. The procedure can be performed using Seldinger or tandem trocar techniques. In the acute setting, ultrasound-guided trocar placement of a locking pigtail catheter can be performed. For conversion of long-term foley catheters to suprapubic tubes, the urinary bladder can be filled with contrast material or saline solution. Then, using ultrasound or fluoroscopy for imaging guidance, an 18-gauge sheathed needle can be advanced into the urinary bladder. The needle position within the bladder is confirmed by gentle aspiration of urine and is followed by placement of a stiff guidewire within the urinary bladder. The sheath is then removed and the percutaneous tract is dilated to the desired catheter size. This can then be delivered into the bladder through a peel-away sheath [18].

Alternatively, trocar placement of a drainage catheter can be easily performed under direct ultrasound or fluoroscopic guidance [19, 20]. Either locking pigtail catheters or Foley catheters mounted on a trocar device are suitable for this technique. The procedure is associated with few complications and usually involves bleeding at the puncture site and urinary sepsis.

References

1. Dyer RB, Regan JD, Kavanagh PV, Khatod EG, Chen MY, Zagoria RJ. Percutaneous nephrostomy with extensions of the technique: step by step. Radiographics: a review publication of the Radiological Society of North America, Inc. 2002;22: 503–25.
2. Ekici S, Sahin A, Ozen H. Percutaneous nephrostomy in the management of malignant ureteral obstruction secondary to bladder cancer. J Endourol. 2001;15:827–9.
3. Cochran S, Barbaric Z, Lee JJ, Kashfian P. Percutaneous nephrostomy tube placement: an outpatient procedure? Radiology. 1991;179:843–7.
4. Spies JB, Rosen R, Lebowitz A. Antibiotic prophylaxis in vascular and interventional radiology: a rational approach. Radiology. 1988;166:381–7.
5. Stone H. Basic principles in the use of prophylactic antibiotics. J Antimicrob Chemother. 1984;14:33–7.
6. Miller NL, Matlaga BR, Lingeman JE. Techniques for fluoroscopic percutaneous renal access. J Urol. 2007;178:15–23.
7. Matlaga BR, Shah OD, Zagoria RJ, Dyer RB, Streem SB, Assimos DG. Computerized tomography guided access for percutaneous nephrostolithotomy. J Urol. 2003;170:45–7.
8. Osman M, Wendt-Nordahl G, Heger K, Michel MS, Alken P, Knoll T. Percutaneous nephrolithotomy with ultrasonography-guided renal access: experience from over 300 cases. BJU Int. 2005;96:875–8.
9. Thanos L, Mylona S, Stroumpouli E, Kalioras V, Pomoni M, Batakis N. Percutaneous CT-guided nephrostomy: a safe and quick alternative method in management of obstructive and non-obstructive uropathy. J Endourol. 2006;20:486–90.

10. Patel U, Hussain F. Percutaneous nephrostomy of nondilated renal collecting systems with fluoroscopic guidance: technique and results. Radiology. 2004;233:226–33.
11. Michel MS, Trojan L, Rassweiler JJ. Complications in percutaneous nephrolithotomy. Eur Urol. 2007;51:899–906. discussion 906.
12. Skolarikos A, De La Rosette J. Prevention and treatment of complications following percutaneous nephrolithotomy. Current opinion in urology. 2008;18:229–34.
13. Cope C, Zeit R. Pseudoaneurysms after nephrostomy. AJR Am J Roentgenol. 1982;139:255–61.
14. Lang E. Percutaneous nephrostolithotomy and lithotripsy: a multi-institutional survey of complications. Radiology. 1987;162:25–30.
15. Leroy A, Williams HJ, Bender C, Segura J, Patterson D, Benson R. Colon perforation following percutaneous nephrostomy and renal calculus removal. Radiology. 1985;155:83–5.
16. Picus D, Weyman P, Clayman R, Mcclennan B. Intercostal-space nephrostomy for percutaneous stone removal. AJR Am J Roentgenol. 1986;147:393–7.
17. Zagoria RJ, Dyer RB. Do's and don't's of percutaneous nephrostomy. Academic radiology. 1999;6:370–7.
18. Papanicolaou N, Pfister RC, Nocks BN. Percutaneous, large-bore, suprapubic cystostomy: technique and results. AJR Am J Roentgenol. 1989;152:303–6.
19. Lawrentschuk N, Lee D, Marriott P, Russell JM. Suprapubic stab cystostomy: a safer technique. Urology. 2003;62:932–4.
20. Lee MJ, Papanicolaou N, Nocks B, Valdez J, Yoder I. Fluoroscopically guided percutaneous suprapubic cystostomy for long-term bladder drainage: an alternative to surgical cystostomy. Radiology. 1993;188:787–9.

5 Percutaneous Gastrostomy and Gastrojejunostomy

Abstract Percutaneous gastrostomy is a safe, low-cost method of providing essential nutrition without the discomfort of a nasogastric tube [1]. The interventional radiologist plays an increasingly important role in the creation and maintenance of enteral access. Of the three standard methods available for gastrostomy (surgical, endoscopic, radiologic), radiologic percutaneous gastrostomy is the least invasive and is associated with less morbidity and mortality when compared to surgical or endoscopic approaches [2, 3]. In many cases, radiologic percutaneous gastrostomy can be performed as an outpatient procedure and feedings can be initiated shortly after placement. For patients at risk of aspiration due to gastroesophageal reflux, percutaneous gastrostomy can be easily converted to percutaneous gastrojejunostomy. Finally, radiologic percutaneous gastrostomy placed under fluoroscopic guidance has been shown to have lower costs when compared to endoscopic and surgical approaches.

Keywords Gastrostomy • Gastrojejunostomy • Gastropexy

Indications

Percutaneous gastrostomy is most frequently indicated for long-term enteral nutrition, typically for patients who are

R.S. Arellano, *Non-Vascular Interventional Radiology of the Abdomen*, DOI 10.1007/978-1-4419-7732-8_5, © Springer Science+Business Media, LLC 2011

unable to eat for extended periods of time. A number of patient populations fall into this category, include those with deglutition abnormalities as a result of neurologic disorders, including stroke, anoxic brain injury, or neurodegenerative disease. Patients with head and neck cancers, eating disorders, or intestinal malabsorption also benefit from percutaneous gastrostomy [4–6]. For this subgroup of patients, percutaneous gastrostomy offers temporary palliation while awaiting restoration of swallowing mechanism or for allowing time for healing of fistulas [7]. Percutaneous gastrostomy can also be used for gastric or bowel decompression [8–10].

Contraindications

Certain anatomic or pathological conditions may increase the risk of percutaneous gastrostomy. Relative contraindications for percutaneous gastrostomy include coagulopathy, unfavorable anatomy, gastric tumor, gastric varices, or active gastritis. Massive ascites had previously been considered to be a relative contraindication to percutaneous gastrostomy. However, with preprocedural paracentesis, gastropexy has been shown to be effective for the successful placement of gastrostomy catheters to reduce the risk of pericatheter leakage and catheter dislodgement.

Catheters

A variety of catheter types can be used for percutaneous gastrostomy, including Foley catheters, pigtail-type locking catheters, endoscopic type catheters, and button catheters. Foley catheters are still common for surgical gastrostomy, but are seldom used for image-guided percutaneous gastrostomy. They remain helpful, however, as a temporary catheter placed through an existing percutaneous tract when other types of gastrostomy tubes inadvertently fall out. Otherwise, the specific type used ultimately depends on user or institutional preferences.

Preprocedural Evaluation

Patients should have an intravenous line for the administration of medications for conscious sedation or anesthesia. Antibiotic prophylaxis has been shown to help minimize the risk of peristomal infection and selection direction toward skin flora should be considered [11–13]. Coagulopathies should be corrected whenever possible. Limited ultrasound examination of the abdomen helps identify the left hepatic lobe and its relationship to the stomach [14, 15]. Gastric distention with air is necessary for the procedure, so placement of a nasogastric tube is essential. This can be placed at the bedside before the patient arrives in radiology. Alternatively, a 5-Fr vascular catheter can be placed under fluoroscopic guidance when the patient arrives in the radiology suite [16]. In rare circumstances where the stomach cannot be distended by these means, CT or US-guided puncture of the stomach with a 20-gauge followed by air insufflations can be used [17]. Giving the patient of barium the evening prior to the procedure (approximately 8 oz.) helps define the relationship of the transverse colon to the stomach [15]. When patients cannot ingest barium, a barium or gastrograffin enema can be performed immediately prior to the procedure. Aside from the ingestion of barium 8 h prior to the procedure, it is generally accepted that patients should be fasting overnight.

Technique

Percutaneous radiologic gastrostomy is performed primarily with the use of fluoroscopic guidance, using Seldinger technique [18–20]. Ultrasound or computed tomography is rarely utilized, except for unusual circumstances [21, 22].

Preliminary fluoroscopy of the unprepared abdomen is performed to identify contrast in the transverse colon. A limited ultrasound examination abdomen can be performed to identify the left hepatic lobe and to make the skin overlying its location so as to avoid puncture during gastropexy. Once the liver and transverse colon have been adequately identified, the stomach is insufflated with air via the nasogastric tube. With the stomach distended, fluoroscopy is used to identify a suitable puncture site on the skin (Fig. 5.1). The mid to distal gastric body is preferred for the placement of the tube [14, 15]. The skin is then infiltrated with local anesthesia. Gastropexy is performed to secure the stomach to the anterior abdominal wall and thus minimize catheter dislodgement and spillage of gastric contents into the peritoneal cavity [23–27]. Gastropexy is performed with the use of a specially manufactured 20-gauge needle that allows the insertion of a metal fastener at the beveled tip. The metal fastener is manufactured with a monofilament suture that is preloaded with a cotton pledgette. The needle is advanced under fluoroscopic guidance into the stomach. Intraluminal position of the needle tip can be confirmed by aspirating air into an attached small syringe. A 0.035" guidewire is then used to push the metal fastener out of the needle and into the gastric lumen (Fig. 5.2). Manual tension is then applied to the attached suture material until the cotton pledgette forms a gentle indentation on the skin. Two aluminum hollow cylinders that are part of the fastener system are then clamped onto the suture with

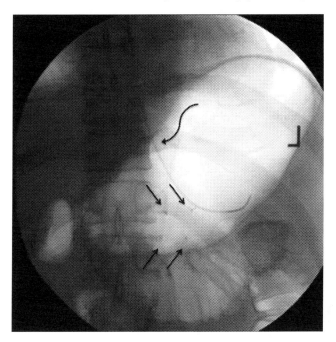

Figure 5.1. *Curved black arrow points* to a nasogastric catheter in the stomach used for insufflation. The *short black arrows points* to four 25-gauge needles placed on the skin to mark the site for gastropexy.

hemostats. These act to keep the fastener secured to the skin and to maintain gentle tension of the stomach against the peritoneal lining.

Once the gastropexy is complete, the stomach is punctured with the 18-gauge needle and a 0.035" guidewire is then advanced into the stomach. Gastric puncture with an angle of entry directed toward the antrum is favored, as this facilitates conversion of a gastrostomy tube for a gastrojejunostomy catheter in those patients who demonstrate significant gastroesophageal reflux. Fascial dilators are then used to dilate the subcutaneous tissues. When a button type catheter is used, an angioplasty balloon is often necessary in

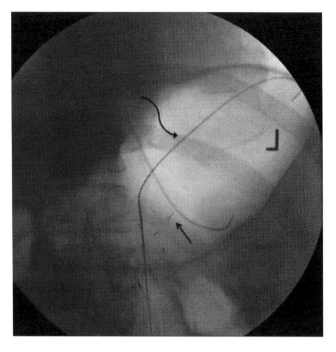

Figure 5.2. The *short black arrow points* to a T-fastener that has been placed into the gastric lumen by a guidewire (*curved white arrow*) that was advanced through an 18-gauge needle.

order to sufficiently dilate the subcutaneous tissue for delivery of the catheter. With the subcutaneous tissues adequately dilated, the gastrostomy catheter can then be delivered into the stomach through a peel away-sheath, with or without a guidewire depending on the type of catheter that is used. Contrast injection confirms intraluminal placement of the catheter (Fig. 5.3). T-fasteners should be removed 7–10 days after placement to allow formation of a subcutaneous tract. Feeding through the gastrostomy is started approximately 12–24 h after procedure. Thorough flushing of the catheter after each feeding is necessary in order to prevent catheter occlusion.

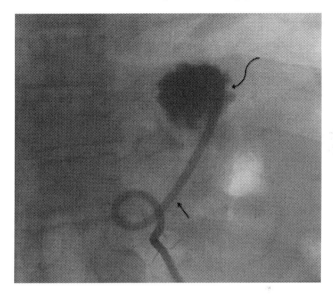

Figure 5.3. Radiography demonstrating final position of the gastrostomy catheter. The *straight arrow points* to the gastrostomy tube. Contrast has been injected through the catheter has opacified the gastric fundus (*curved arrow*), confirming its position within the stomach.

Gastrojejunostomy

Occasionally, primary gastrojejunostomy or conversion of an existing gastrostomy to a gastrojejunostomy is requested. Primary percutaneous gastrojejunostomy is technically similar to percutaneous gastrostomy. Cope-locking gastrojejunostomy catheters have a similar shape to pigtail type catheters but are longer. They are indicated for patients who suffer from significant gastroesophageal reflux who are at risk of aspiration in the setting of a fluid-filled gastric fundus. In contrast to gastrostomy where the catheter tip resides in the fundus, the tip of the gastrojejunostomy catheter is placed into the proximal jejunum. To achieve this, the angle of entry for the gastric puncture is directed toward the antrum, and then the guidewire is negotiated through the pylorus and duodenum to the ligament of Trietz. Tract dilatation is identical to that of percutaneous gastrostomy, and the catheter is then delivered into the small bowel through a peel-away sheath. Conversion of an existing gastrostomy catheter to a gastrojejunostomy catheter should be considered in patients who suffer from significant gastroesophageal reflux. This is facilitated when the initial angle of entry for the gastrostomy tube is directed toward the antrum. To achieve conversion, the stomach is insufflated with air. A guidewire is negotiated through the tube and into the duodenum. This usually requires replacing the gastrostomy catheter with a 5-Fr directional catheter. Once the wire is into the proximal jejunum, the 5-Fr catheter is replaced with the new gastrojejunostomy catheter.

Results

The technical success rates for percutaneous gastrostomy and gastrojejunostomy is reported as high as 95–100% with low complication rates [3, 28–30]. Reported procedure-related complications are less than 5% [1, 3, 31, 32].

Complications

Major complications related to percutaneous gastrostomy include wound infection, aspiration, hemorrhages requiring transfusion, peritonitis, and sepsis have been reported in up to 6% of patients [33–36]. However, most complications are minor and include peritubal leakage, local skin infection, and tube dislodgement [37–39]. In a meta-analysis comparing radiological gastrostomy with endoscopic and surgical gastrostomy, Wollman et al. reported a success rate of 99.2% with mortality <1% [3].

Follow-Up Care

Feeding through gastrostomy catheters can begin 12–24 h after placement. In contrast, gastrojejunostomy catheters can be used immediately. Catheters should be thoroughly flushed after each use in order to reduce the potential for catheter occlusion. Tubes that become inadvertently dislodged can usually be replaced within 24 h after removal. In the acute setting, a Foley catheter can often be placed into the stomach, as long as the subcutaneous tract remains open. The catheter position should then be confirmed radiographically before feeding through the tube is begun. When the subcutaneous tract has healed, a new primary puncture is often necessary.

Conclusion

Percutaneous radiologic gastrostomy and gastrojejunostomy are effective and safe procedures that are technically easy to perform. They are associated with low morbidity and mortality rates. In most cases, they can be performed with the use of procedural sedation, require short hospitalization and in selected cases can be performed as outpatient procedures.

References

1. Ho CS, Gray R, Goldfinger M, Rosen I, Mcpherson R. Percutaneous gastrostomy for enteral feeding. Radiology. 1985;156:349–51.
2. O'Dwyer TP, Gullane P, Awerbuch D, Ho CS. Percutaneous feeding gastrostomy in patients with head and neck tumors: a 5-year review. Laryngoscope. 1990;100:29–32.
3. Cady J. Nutritional support during radiotherapy for head and neck cancer: the role of prophylactic feeding tube placement. Clin J Oncol Nurs. 2007;11:875–80.

4. Myssiorek D, Siegel D, Vambutas A. Fluoroscopically placed percutaneous gastrostomies in the head and neck patient. Laryngoscope. 1998;108:1557–60.

5. Grassi CJ. Modified gastrojejunostomy tube: percutaneous placement for gastric decompression and jejunal feeding. Radiology. 1989;173:875–6.

6. O'Keeffe F, Carrasco C, Charnsangavej C, Richli W, Wallace S, Freedman R. Percutaneous drainage and feeding gastrostomies in 100 patients. Radiology. 1989;172:341–3.

7. Hicks M, Surratt R, Picus D, Marx M, Lang E. Fluoroscopically guided percutaneous gastrostomy and gastroenterostomy: analysis of 158 consecutive cases. AJR Am J Roentgenol. 1990;154:725–8.

8. Dormann A, Wigginghaus B, Risius H, Kleimann F, Kloppenborg A, Grunewald T, et al. A single dose of ceftriaxone administered 30 minutes before percutaneous endoscopic gastrostomy significantly reduces local and systemic infective complications. Am J Gastroenterol. 1999;94:3220–4.

9. Sane S, Towbin A, Bergey E, Kaye R, Fitz C, Albright L, et al. Percutaneous gastrostomy tube placement in patients with ventriculoperitoneal shunts. Pediatr Radiol. 1998;28:521–3.

10. Cantwell C, Perumpillichira JJ, Maher M, Hahn P, Arellano R, Gervais D, et al. Antibiotic prophylaxis for percutaneous radiologic gastrostomy and gastrojejunostomy insertion in outpatients with head and neck cancer. J Vasc Interv Radiol. 2008;19:571–5.

11. Wills J, Oglesby J. Percutaneous gastrostomy. Radiology. 1983;149:449–53.

12. Brown A, Mueller P, Ferrucci JJ. Controlled percutaneous gastrostomy: nylon T-fastener for fixation of the anterior gastric wall. Radiology. 1986;158:543–5.

13. Wills J, Oglesby J. Percutaneous gastrostomy: further experience. Radiology. 1985;154:71–4.

14. Brady A. Percutaneous gastrostomy: US guidance for gastric puncture. Radiology. 2000;214:303–4.

15. Saini S, Mueller P, Gaa J, Briggs S, Hahn P, Forman B, et al. Percutaneous gastrostomy with gastropexy: experience in 125 patients. AJR Am J Roentgenol. 1990;154:1003–6.

16. Cosentini E, Sautner T, Gnant M, Winkelbauer F, Teleky B, Jakesz R. Outcomes of surgical, percutaneous endoscopic, and percutaneous radiologic gastrostomies. Arch Surg. 1998;133:1076–83.

17. Shin K, Shin J, Song H, Yang Z, Kim JH, Kim KR. Primary and conversion percutaneous gastrojejunostomy under fluoroscopic guidance: 10 years of experience. Clin Imaging. 2008;32: 274–9.
18. Sanchez R, Vansonnenberg E, D'Agostino HB, Goodacre B, Moyers P, Casola G. CT guidance for percutaneous gastrostomy and gastroenterostomy. Radiology. 1992;184:201–5.
19. Hoffer E. US-guided percutaneous gastrostomy: a portable technique. J Vasc Interv Radiol. 1996;7:431–4.
20. De Baere T, Chapot R, Kuoch V, Chevallier P, Delille J, Domenge C, et al. Percutaneous gastrostomy with fluoroscopic guidance: single-center experience in 500 consecutive cancer patients. Radiology. 1999;210:651–4.
21. Qanadli S, Barre O, Mesurolle B, El HM, Mulot R, Strumza P, et al. Percutaneous gastrostomy for enteral nutrition: long-term follow-up of 176 procedures. Can Assoc Radiol J. 1999;50:260–4.
22. Dewald C, Hiette P, Sewall L, Fredenberg P, Palestrant A. Percutaneous gastrostomy and gastrojejunostomy with gastropexy: experience in 701 procedures. Radiology. 1999;211:651–6.
23. Thornton F, Fotheringham T, Haslam P, Mcgrath F, Keeling F, Lee MJ. Percutaneous radiologic gastrostomy with and without T-fastener gastropexy: a randomized comparison study. Cardiovasc Intervent Radiol. 2002;25:467–71.
24. Ryan J, Hahn P, Boland G, Mcdowell R, Saini S, Mueller P. Percutaneous gastrostomy with T-fastener gastropexy: results of 316 consecutive procedures. Radiology. 1997;203:496–500.
25. Wollman B, D'Agostino HB, Walus-Wigle JR, Easter D, Beale A. Radiologic, endoscopic, and surgical gastrostomy: an institutional evaluation and meta-analysis of the literature. Radiology. 1995;197:699–704.
26. Bell S. Cost of performing a radiologic percutaneous gastrostomy. Radiology. 1996;200:586.
27. Cwikiel W, Walther B. Simplified percutaneous gastrostomy. Acta Radiol. 1996;37:535–8.
28. Wollman B, D'Agostino HB. Percutaneous radiologic and endoscopic gastrostomy: a 3-year institutional analysis of procedure performance. AJR Am J Roentgenol. 1997;169:1551–3.
29. Cozzi G, Gavazzi C, Civelli E, Milella M, Salvetti M, Scaperrotta G, et al. Percutaneous gastrostomy in oncologic patients: analysis of results and expansion of the indications. Abdom Imaging. 2000;25:239–42.

30. Lu DS, Mueller P, Lee MJ, Dawson S, Hahn P, Brountzos E. Gastrostomy conversion to transgastric jejunostomy: technical problems, causes of failure, and proposed solutions in 63 patients. Radiology. 1993;187:679–83.
31. Moller P, Lindberg C, Zilling T. Gastrostomy by various techniques: evaluation of indications, outcome, and complications. Scand J Gastroenterol. 1999;34:1050–4.
32. Wills J. Percutaneous gastrostomy: applications in gastric carcinoma and gastroplasty stoma dilatation. AJR Am J Roentgenol. 1986;147:826–7.
33. Rose D, Wolman S, Ho CS. Gastric hemorrhage complicating percutaneous transgastric jejunostomy. Radiology. 1986;161:835–6.
34. Sy K, Dipchand A, Atenafu E, Chait P, Bannister L, Temple M, et al. Safety and effectiveness of radiologic percutaneous gastrostomy and gastro jejunostomy in children with cardiac disease. AJR Am J Roentgenol. 2008;191:1169–74.
35. Gray R, St Louis EL, Grosman H. Percutaneous gastrostomy and gastro-jejunostomy. Br J Radiol. 1987;60:1067–70.
36. Alley J, Corneille M, Stewart R, Dent D. Pneumoperitoneum after percutaneous endoscopic gastrostomy in patients in the intensive care unit. Am Surg. 2007;73:765–7. discussion 768.
37. Wojtowycz M, Arata JJ. Subcutaneous emphysema after percutaneous gastrostomy. AJR Am J Roentgenol. 1988;151:311–2.
38. Gray R, St Louis EL, Grosman H. Modified catheter for percutaneous gastrojejunostomy. Radiology. 1989;173:276–8.
39. Ho CS, Yee AC, Mcpherson R. Complications of surgical and percutaneous nonendoscopic gastrostomy: review of 233 patients. Gastroenterology. 1988;95:1206–10.

6 Biliary Interventions

Abstract Biliary obstruction can result from various factors, including tumors arising from the bile ducts, the liver or adjacent structures such as pancreatic or gastric tumors and metastatic lymphadenopathy. When severe, biliary obstruction negatively impairs the quality of life, usually from symptoms of pruritis, not to mention the risk of cholangitis and sepsis. For these patients, percutaneous cholangiography is useful to help define the point and/or cause of obstruction. Percutaneous drainage of the biliary tree also offers palliation from the devastating symptoms of obstruction.

Keywords Biliary obstruction • Transhepatic cholangiogram • Percutaneous drainage • Cholecystostomy

Percutaneous Transhepatic Cholangiography

Image-guided percutaneous transhepatic cholangiography and drainage are safe and effective techniques that are used to diagnose and treat biliary abnormalities. Percutaneous transhepatic cholangiography involves imaging-guided placement of a 21-gauge or smaller needle into peripheral biliary radicals, followed by injection of contrast material

R.S. Arellano, *Non-Vascular Interventional Radiology of the Abdomen*, DOI 10.1007/978-1-4419-7732-8_6, © Springer Science+Business Media, LLC 2011

into the biliary tree. Successful percutaneous transhepatic cholangiography includes adequate needle placement within the biliary tree and opacification with contrast to allow diagnosis or treatment planning.

Indications for Transhepatic Cholangiography

It is used to define levels of obstruction in patients with biliary dilatation, to evaluate for suspected choledocholithiasis, to evaluate inflammatory conditions of the bile ducts, to assess for the etiology of cholangitis, to define sites of biliary leakage. In transplant patients, it can be used to assess dysfunction of the transplanted hepatic graft.

Percutaneous transhepatic biliary drainage is the next logical step following transhepatic cholangiography. Transhepatic cholangiography provides a "roadmap" for subsequent guidewire manipulations and that ultimately lead to catheter drainage. It can be used as either a primary or palliative method to treat biliary tract abnormalities but may also be the initial step of staged procedures, such as balloon dilatation of anastomotic strictures, brush biopsy, or placement of endoprostheses.

Indications for Percutaneous Biliary Drainage

Indications for percutaneous transhepatic drainage include decompression of an obstructed biliary tree and to provide adequate drainage, to provide access to the biliary system for therapeutic or diagnostic procedures, including dilation of biliary strictures, stone extraction, placement of metal endoprostheses, brachytherapy, and transhepatic biliary brush biopsy [1–4].

Contraindications

Coagulopathy is a relative contraindication to percutaneous biliary procedures, including transhepatic cholangiography and biliary drainage. Careful review of coagulation profiles and efforts to correct or improve coagulapathies should be undertaken whenever possible before the procedure. Patients with partially corrected coagulopathies may still undergo these procedures when absolutely indicated when the morbidity of the procedure is less than that of alternative methods.

Imaging Guidance

Imaging-guided percutaneous access to the biliary tree is routinely achieved with ultrasound or fluoroscopy [5–7]. Magnetic resonance imaging is technically feasible, but not practical [8]. Ultrasound offers the benefits of real-time imaging of needle placement directly into the ducts. It can be used for access to the left or right ducts [7].

Technique

Percutaneous cholangiography and biliary drainages involve at least a moderate amount of discomfort, especially during tract dilatation and when crossing strictures. These procedures should therefore be performed with intravenous conscious sedation and/or general anesthesia, depending on the overall patient condition comorbidities [9–12]. Patients should also receive preprocedure intravenous antibiotics, with medications selected for gram-negative coverage.

Patients are placed supine on the fluoroscopy table. For right-sided punctures, the right arm placed can be placed above the head to allow unrestricted access to the right midaxillary line. For left-sided punctures, the arms are maintained at the sides. A sterile field is prepared at the proposed skin puncture site and the skin, subcutaneous tissues and hepatic capsule are infiltrated with local anesthesia. When ultrasound is used, a peripherally located biliary radical is punctured and is used to obtain a cholangiogram that is then used for a secondary puncture into the biliary system. Alternatively, when only fluoroscopic guidance is used, the liver is punctured with a coaxial needle at the level of the right midaxillary line and directed slightly anteriorly toward the T10 vertebral body. The inner styllette is then withdrawn and a contrast material-filled syringe is attached. While the needle is slowly withdrawn, small amounts of contrast material are injected until a duct is entered. A bile sample is removed for analysis and then additional contrast is injected to opacify the biliary tree to the level of the obstruction. Left-sided access to the biliary tree is frequently performed with the use of ultrasound guidance [7, 13]. This approach is especially useful when the left hepatic lobe extends well below the xiphoid process of the sternum. The left-sided ducts of the left lobe in this location are often within a few centimeters of the skin. Typically, the segment II duct follows a more linear course to the common bile duct, which in turn facilitates guidewire and catheter manipulations.

Initial puncture of the biliary tree is accomplished using a 21- to 22-gauge CHIBA (Cook, Inc., Bloomington, IN) needle or with an 18-gauge-sheathed needle Fig. 6.1. If the CHIBA needle has entered a duct that is suitable for drainage, the inner styllette is removed and exchanged for a 0.018" guidewire. The guidewire should be advanced a sufficient distance within the biliary tree such that the stainless steel component of the guidewire is secured within the duct. The CHIBA needle is then exchanged over the guidewire for a sheath/dilator system that allows placement of a 0.038" working guidewire.

When the initial access into the biliary tree with the CHIBA needle is unsuitable for drainage, this needle is then used to opacify the ducts for secondary puncture for a more favorable duct. This is accomplished with either a second 21- or 22-gauge CHIBA needle with a sheathed 18-gauge needle. The benefit of performing the secondary puncture with the sheathed needle is that it eliminates the need for upsizing from a 0.018" to a larger working wire. When a suitable duct for drainage is identified, a 0.035"–0.038" 3-J floppy tipped guidewire is then advanced into the biliary tree and negotiated across the site of obstruction and ultimately into the duodenum. At this point, the 3-J floppy wire is exchanged for a stiffer working wire. The puncture site and transhepatic path to the entered bile duct is then dilated using fascial dilators. A dilator/peel-away sheath system is then advanced over the guidewire into the bile duct. The dilator is removed and replaced with a multi-side-hole drainage catheter. The catheter should be positioned such that the side holes are located proximal and distal to the site of the obstruction [14] (Fig. 6.1).

Care should be taken to limit the manipulations of the biliary tree with guidewires and catheters when attempting to negotiate across biliary obstructions in order to minimize the risk of acute biliary sepsis. This is especially relevant for patients with suppurative cholangitis in whom manipulations should be held to a minimum. In most instances, 5–10 min of gentle probing with the guidewire and catheter is sufficient time to attempt to cross a point of obstruction. When this fails, the biliary system should be decompressed with external drainage for 2–3 days. Repeated attempts to

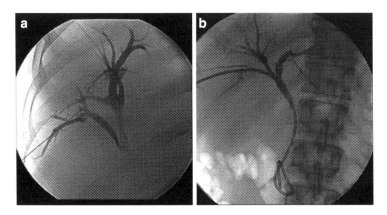

Figure 6.1. (**a**) Transhepatic cholangiogram demonstrating opacification of the biliary tree from a right posterior duct access. (**b**) Fluoroscopic image demonstrating final position of percutaneous biliary catheter.

cross the biliary tree at a later time are frequently successful and in many cases safer for the patient.

Once the catheter is satisfactorily positioned within the biliary system, it is held in place by the locking pigtail tip and then secured at the level of the skin with a retention device. The catheter is connected via drainage tube to a receptacle for gravity drainage. Drainage catheters should be flushed at least two to three times per day with approximately 10 mL of normal saline solution to ensure patency. For long-term biliary percutaneous biliary drainage, catheters should be exchanged on a regularly scheduled basis, typically every 4–8 weeks in order to prevent occlusion.

Several types of biliary drainage can be achieved once the biliary tree has been accessed. In *external biliary drainage*, the catheter side holes are positioned proximal to the site of obstruction, and all biliary drainage is diverted externally via the catheter. This type of drainage is necessary for patients with suppurative cholangitis in whom attempts to cross the point of biliary obstruction should be kept to a minimum. Attempts to cross the point of biliary obstruction can be undertaken once the patient's overall medical condition improves. Alternatively, external biliary drainage may be the only option for long-standing or complete biliary obstruction that precludes traversing with a catheter. While effective, external biliary drainage is prone to catheter dislodgement due to its relative insecure position with the biliary tree.

For *internal/external biliary drainage*, the catheter traverses the point of obstruction and in contrast to external biliary drainage, the locking pigtail distal to the point of obstruction helps to maintain catheter position within the biliary tree. Internal/external drainage allows bile to be diverted internally as well as externally. Catheter exchanges, when necessary are easily accomplished over a guidewire and the external conduit to the biliary tree and small bowel provides access for a number of other procedures, such as placement of a metal stent or brachytherapy.

Complications

Complications related to percutaneous biliary interventions are classified as procedure-related and late complications. Procedure-related complications include adverse reactions to sedation, hemorrhage, pleural effusions, biloma, or biliary sepsis [15–19].

Percutaneous Management of Benign Biliary Strictures

Careful patient selection is necessary to determine whether or not percutaneous management of biliary strictures is indicated. Treatment planning for benign biliary strictures hinges upon the availability of alternative treatment options and the likelihood that benign strictures will recur. Typical patients with benign strictures include those caused by nonanastomotic narrowing postliver transplant, posthepaticojejunostomy, and sclerosing cholangitis [20–23]. Because of the benign nature of these types of strictures and the long life expectancy of these patients, placement of metal stents is usually discouraged, unless the patient has a short life expectancy for other causes or is being considered for liver transplantation.

Transluminal angioplasty balloons are used to dilate benign strictures. These are placed within the biliary tree via the access route established by percutaneous internal/external drainage. As with primary biliary drainage, balloon angioplasty of benign strictures can be very painful, and this procedure should be undertaken with deep conscious sedation or general anesthesia.

Technical success for dilatation of benign strictures is reported as high as 90–100% [24–26]. Long-term patency rates vary depending on the nature of the stricture and can range from 42 to 76% Iatrogenic strictures tend to have response rates of >70% [27–29].

Management of Malignant Biliary Strictures

In contrast to patients with benign strictures, expandable metallic stents may be indicated for patients with malignant obstruction in whom the patency of the stent is expected to exceed the life expectancy of the patient [30–34]. When compared to plastic stents, metallic stents tend to remain patent for longer periods of time, are less prone to complications and require fewer stent revisions to maintain patency.

Percutaneous Cholecystostomy

Cholecystectomy is the preferred method of treatment for acute calculous cholecystitis [35]. While cholecystectomy is a relatively safe procedure, the morbidity and mortality of the procedure can be as high as 30% for patients who are severely ill or elderly [36–38]. For these patients, as well as those with acalculous cholecystitis, image-guided percutaneous cholecystostomy offers an alternative or temporizing treatment option [39, 40]. Percutaneous cholecystostomy allows immediate decompression of the inflamed gallbladder with rapid resolution of symptoms [41]. Percutaneous cholecystostomy can be followed by elective cholecystectomy when the underlying condition improves, as soon as the patient stabilizes and no sepsis is present, or by conservative management in high surgical-risk patients [42]. The technical success rate for percutaneous cholecystostomy has been reported as high as 100% with clinical success as high as 91% and is associated with few complications [43]. Bleeding, bile leak/biloma and bile peritonitis have been reported as complications of this procedure, but the overall complication rate is low. Percutaneous cholecystostomy may be the only treatment necessary for acalculous cholecystitis.

Indications

While percutaneous cholecystostomy is one means of providing access to the biliary system for a number of biliary interventions, its primary role is for the decompression of an acutely inflamed gallbladder. The diagnosis of acute cholecystitis is usually suspected in the setting of right upper quadrant pain, fever, and leukocystosis. Sonographic features that support the diagnosis of acute cholecystitis include gallstones (for calculous cholecystitis), gallbladder wall thickening greater than 3 mm, pericholecystic fluid, gallbladder distention, and the sonographic Murphy's sign. The presence of these findings in the absence of gallstones should raise the possibility of acalculous cholecystitis, a condition that is frequently encountered in intensive care unit patients or those receiving total parenteral nutrition.

Technique

Percutaneous cholecystostomy can be performed with intravenous sedation and local anesthesia after initiation of intravenous antibiotic coverage. Coagulopathies should be corrected with fresh frozen plasma or platelets, or both, as clinically indicated. Percutaneous cholecystostomy is typically performed using ultrasound guidance, though it can also be performed using combined ultrasound and fluoroscopic or computed tomography guidance [44, 45]. Ultrasonography allows precise puncture of the gall bladder during real time imaging and offers the added benefit of performing the procedure portably at the bedside [46].

The gallbladder is punctured using either a transperitoneal and transhepatic approach. Both approaches are similar in short-term safety and show no real significant difference in terms of complication rates for either approach [47–49]. However, the transhepatic approach may be preferred in the absence of severe hepatic disease or coagulopathies [50, 51] because of the theoretical benefit of stability of the catheter within the liver parenchyma [49] that may decrease the risk of bile peritonitis. Transperitoneal approach may be considered when minimal trauma to the hepatic parenchyma is preferred in order to minimize the risk of hemorrhage or infectious complications in the setting of severe hepatic disease or coagulopathies.

Percutaneous cholecystostomy can be performed using either the trocar method or with Seldinger technique. With the trocar method, ultrasound guidance is used to identify the gallbladder. Using a locking pigtail catheter mounted on a trocar needle, the gallbladder is punctured under direct ultrasound guidance (Fig. 6.2). Once the catheter tip is within the gallbladder lumen, it is released from the trocar needle and advanced into the gallbladder.

With Seldinger technique, the gallbladder is punctured with an 18-gauge needle or 22-20 gauge needle that accepts a 0.018" guidewire. Once the lumen is accessed and a guidewire has been placed within the gallbladder, the access route is expanded with fascial dilators and a locking pigtail catheter is advanced over the guidewire into the gallbladder lumen.

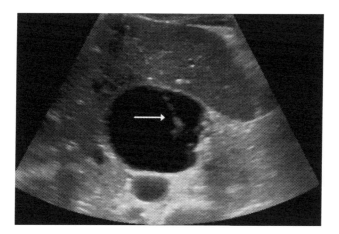

Figure 6.2. Ultrasound image of the gallbladder that demonstrates percutaneous placement of a drainage catheter (*white arrow*) into the gallbladder lumen.

Bile specimens should be sent for microbiological testing and the gallbladder should be fully decompressed. Flushing the gallbladder with saline at the time of initial drainage should be discouraged as over manipulation of the gallbladder may encourage sepsis [52]. When fluoroscopic guidance is used for drainage, a small amount of contrast can be injected to confirm catheter position. Thereafter, the catheter is secured to the skin with a retention device and connected to a drainage bag for gravity drainage.

Follow-Up

Imaging of the percutaneous tract is necessary to assess for adequacy of catheter removal [53]. Catheters should be removed only if a well-granulated tract has formed between the gallbladder and skin. It has been suggested that approximately 3 weeks time is necessary for tracts to form. Removal of catheters from incompletely formed tracts can result in bile peritonitis and acute pain that require emergent surgery. The catheter is removed over a guidewire and is replaced with an angiographic catheter of similar size. The tract is injected with contrast. If there is a continuous tract from the gallbladder to the skin without evidence of leakage of contrast into the peritoneal space (Fig. 6.3), the catheter is removed. The catheter is replaced when contrast injection of the tract show leakage into the peritoneal space.

Tract maturation is an integral component of percutaneous cholecystostomy and is essential to minimize the risk of bile leakage and subsequent peritonitis. It is generally accepted that approximately 3 weeks are necessary to allow maturation of the percutaneous tract for either transhepatic or transperitoneal approaches. This time frame may be extended with patients with severe underlying medical conditions, such as diabetes mellitus, chronic steroid use, or

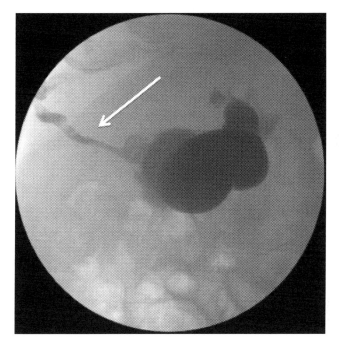

Figure 6.3. Fluoroscopic image demonstrating contrast injection through an existing transhepatic cholecystostomy tract (*white arrow*). The transhepatic tract should extend to the skin and show no evidence of spillage into the peritoneal cavity before the catheter is completely removed. An incompletely formed tract that spills bile into the peritoneal cavity can result in painful bile peritonitis.

chronic renal failure [54, 55]. Catheter removal should not be undertaken until a well-established tract has formed. Maturation of the tract can be assessed by injection of contrast through the tract. To accomplish this, the catheter is removed over a guidewire under fluoroscopic guidance and replaced with a 5-Fr angiographic catheter. Contrast is injected through the catheter as it is slowly withdrawn. The percutaneous cholecystostomy catheter should be replaced if the contrast injection shows any evidence of spillage into the peritoneal space. However, not all patients may require tube injection as an antecedent step toward removal. Wise et al. showed that when the cystic and common bile ducts were patent as determined by cholangiography, the catheters could be safely removed without increased risk of bile peritonitis.

Complications

Complications related to percutaneous cholecystostomy usually occur immediately at the time of placement or as delayed complications within days of the procedure. Reported complications include hemorrhage, biliary sepsis, bowel perforation, bile peritonitis, or biloma [48, 50, 56]. Catheter dislodgement is a common late complication. Therefore, premature catheter removal by dislodgement should be replaced to minimize the risk of bile leakage and peritonitis.

References

1. Mendez GJ, Russell E, Levi J, Koolpe H, Cohen M. Percutaneous brush biopsy and internal drainage of biliary tree through endoprosthesis. AJR Am J Roentgenol. 1980;134:653–9.
2. Pugliese V, Barone D, Saccomanno S, Conio M, Aste H, Santi L. Tissue sampling from the common bile duct through endoscopic retrograde cholangiopancreatography, endoscopic papillo (sphinctero)tomy and drainage in juxtapapillary malignancies. Surg Endosc. 1987;1:83–7.
3. Rossi M, Cantisani V, Salvatori F, Rebonato A, Greco L, Giglio L, et al. Histologic assessment of biliary obstruction with different percutaneous endoluminal techniques. BMC Med Imaging. 2004;4:3.
4. Xing G, Geng J, Han XW, Dai JH, Wu CY. Endobiliary brush cytology during percutaneous transhepatic cholangiodrainage in patients with obstructive jaundice. Hepatobiliary Pancreat Dis Int. 2005;4:98–103.

5. Makuuchi M, Yamazaki S, Hasegawa H, Bandai Y, Ito T, Watanabe G. Ultrasonically guided cholangiography and bile drainage. Ultrasound Med Biol. 1984;10:617–23.

6. Lee W, Kim GC, Kim JY, Baik S, Lee HJ, Kim HJ, et al. Ultrasound and fluoroscopy guided percutaneous transhepatic biliary drainage in patients with nondilated bile ducts. Abdom Imaging. 2008;33:555–9.

7. Lameris J, Obertop H, Jeekel J. Biliary drainage by ultrasound-guided puncture of the left hepatic duct. Clin Radiol. 1985;36: 269–74.

8. Wacker F, Faiss S, Reither K, Zimmer T, Wendt M, Wolf K. MR imaging-guided biliary drainage in an open low-field system: first clinical experiences. Rofo. 2000;172:744–7.

9. Trotteur G, Stockx L, Dondelinger R. Sedation, analgesia and anesthesia for interventional radiological procedures in adults. Part I. Survey of interventional radiological practice in Belgium. JBR-BTR. 2000;83:111–5.

10. Lee MJ, Mueller P, Saini S, Hahn P, Dawson S. Percutaneous dilatation of benign biliary strictures: single-session therapy with general anesthesia. AJR Am J Roentgenol. 1991;157: 1263–6.

11. Hatzidakis A, Charonitakis E, Athanasiou A, Tsetis D, Chlouverakis G, Papamastorakis G, et al. Sedations and analgesia in patients undergoing percutaneous transhepatic biliary drainage. Clin Radiol. 2003;58:121–7.

12. Covey AM, Brown K. Percutaneous transhepatic biliary drainage. Tech Vasc Interv Radiol. 2008;11:14–20.

13. Barth K. Percutaneous biliary drainage for high obstruction. Radiol Clin North Am. 1990;28:1223–35.

14. Ring E, Husted J, Oleaga J, Freiman D. A multihole catheter for maintaining longterm percutaneous antegrade biliary drainage. Radiology. 1979;132:752–4.

15. Berquist T, May GR, Johnson C, Adson M, Thistle J. Percutaneous biliary decompression: internal and external drainage in 50 patients. AJR Am J Roentgenol. 1981;136:901–6.

16. Clouse ME, Evans D, Costello P, Alday M, Edwards S, Mcdermott WJ. Percutaneous transhepatic biliary drainage. Complications due to multiple duct obstructions. Ann Surg. 1983;198:25–9.

17. Hamlin J, Friedman M, Stein M, Bray J. Percutaneous biliary drainage: complications of 118 consecutive catheterizations. Radiology. 1986;158:199–202.

18. Yee AC, Ho CS. Complications of percutaneous biliary drainage: benign vs. malignant diseases. AJR Am J Roentgenol. 1987;148: 1207–9.
19. Gunther R, Schild H, Thelen M. Percutaneous transhepatic biliary drainage: experience with 311 procedures. Cardiovasc Intervent Radiol. 1988;11:65–71.
20. Trambert J, Bron K, Zajko A, Starzl T, Iwatsuki S. Percutaneous transhepatic balloon dilatation of benign biliary strictures. AJR Am J Roentgenol. 1987;149:945–8.
21. Schwarz W, Rosen R, Fitts WJ, Mackie J, Oleaga J, Freiman D, et al. Percutaneous transhepatic drainage preoperatively for benign biliary strictures. Surg Gynecol Obstet. 1981;152: 466–8.
22. Morrison M, Lee MJ, Saini S, Brink J, Mueller P. Percutaneous balloon dilatation of benign biliary strictures. Radiol Clin North Am. 1990;28:1191–201.
23. Ko GY, Sung K, Yoon H, Kim KR, Gwon D, Lee SG. Percutaneous transhepatic treatment of hepaticojejunal anastomotic biliary strictures after living donor liver transplantation. Liver Transpl. 2008;14:1323–32.
24. Schumacher B, Othman T, Jansen M, Preiss C, Neuhaus H. Long-term follow-up of percutaneous transhepatic therapy (PTT) in patients with definite benign anastomotic strictures after hepaticojejunostomy. Endoscopy. 2001;33:409–15.
25. Eickhoff A, Schilling D, Jakobs R, Weickert U, Hartmann D, Eickhoff J, et al. Long-term outcome of percutaneous transhepatic drainage for benign bile duct stenoses. Rocz Akad Med Bialymst. 2005;50:155–60.
26. Weber A, Rosca B, Neu B, Rosch T, Frimberger E, Born P, et al. Long-term follow-up of percutaneous transhepatic biliary drainage (PTBD) in patients with benign bilioenterostomy stricture. Endoscopy. 2009;41:323–8.
27. Mueller P, Vansonnenberg E, Ferrucci JJ, Weyman P, Butch R, Malt R, et al. Biliary stricture dilatation: multicenter review of clinical management in 73 patients. Radiology. 1986;160: 17–22.
28. Venbrux A, Osterman FJ. Percutaneous management of benign biliary strictures. Tech Vasc Interv Radiol. 2001;4:141–6.
29. Kocher M, Cerna M, Havlik R, Kral V, Gryga A, Duda M. Percutaneous treatment of benign bile duct strictures. Eur J Radiol. 2007;62:170–4.

30. Kauffmann G, Roeren T, Friedl P, Brambs H, Richter G. Interventional radiological treatment of malignant biliary obstruction. Eur J Surg Oncol. 1990;16:397–403.
31. Laberge J, Doherty M, Gordon R, Ring E. Hilar malignancy: treatment with an expandable metallic transhepatic biliary stent. Radiology. 1990;177:793–7.
32. Glattli A, Stain S, Baer H, Schweizer W, Triller J, Blumgart L. Unresectable malignant biliary obstruction: treatment by self-expandable biliary endoprostheses. HPB Surg. 1993;6:175–84.
33. Tokunaga Y, Mukaihara S, Kubo S, Yang S, Yo M, Nakayama H, et al. Metallic expanding biliary stents in malignant obstruction. Cases with stent in stent. J Clin Gastroenterol. 1993;17: 153–7.
34. Ridtitid W, Rerknimitr R, Janchai A, Kongkam P, Treeprasertsuk S, Kullavanijaya P. Outcome of second interventions for occluded metallic stents in patients with malignant biliary obstruction. Surg Endosc. 2010;24:2216–20.
35. Pickleman J, Gonzalez R. The improving results of cholecystectomy. Arch Surg. 1986;121:930–4.
36. Saito A, Shirai Y, Ohzeki H, Hayashi J, Eguchi S. Acute acalculous cholecystitis after cardiovascular surgery. Surg Today. 1997;27:907–9.
37. Frazee R, Nagorney D, Mucha PJ. Acute acalculous cholecystitis. Mayo Clin Proc. 1989;64:163–7.
38. Li JC, Lee DW, Lai CW, Li AC, Chu DW, Chan A. Percutaneous cholecystostomy for the treatment of acute cholecystitis in the critically ill and elderly. Hong Kong Med J. 2004;10: 389–93.
39. Mcloughlin R, Patterson E, Mathieson J, Cooperberg P, Macfarlane J. Radiologically guided percutaneous cholecystostomy for acute cholecystitis: long-term outcome in 50 patients. Can Assoc Radiol J. 1994;45:455–9.
40. Ginat D, Saad W. Cholecystostomy and transcholecystic biliary access. Tech Vasc Interv Radiol. 2008;11:2–13.
41. Eggermont A, Lameris J, Jeekel J. Ultrasound-guided percutaneous transhepatic cholecystostomy for acute acalculous cholecystitis. Arch Surg. 1985;120:1354–6.
42. Berman M, Nudelman I, Fuko Z, Madhala O, Neuman-Levin M, Lelcuk S. Percutaneous transhepatic cholecystostomy: effective treatment of acute cholecystitis in high risk patients. Isr Med Assoc J. 2002;4:331–3.

43. Ha JP, Tsui K, Tang C, Siu WT, Fung K, Li MK. Cholecystectomy or not after percutaneous cholecystostomy for acute calculous cholecystitis in high-risk patients. Hepatogastroenterology. 2008;55:1497–502.

44. Mcgahan J, Anderson M, Walter J. Portable real-time sonographic and needle guidance systems for aspiration and drainage. AJR Am J Roentgenol. 1986;147:1241–6.

45. Wise J, Gervais D, Akman A, Harisinghani M, Hahn P, Mueller P. Percutaneous cholecystostomy catheter removal and incidence of clinically significant bile leaks: a clinical approach to catheter management. AJR Am J Roentgenol. 2005;184: 1647–51.

46. Dunham F, Marliere P, Mortier C, Gulbis A. Ultrasound-guided percutaneous and transhepatic cholecystostomy: a complementary procedure to therapeutic endoscopy. Endoscopy. 1985;17: 153–6.

47. Loberant N, Notes Y, Eitan A, Yakir O, Bickel A. Comparison of early outcome from transperitoneal versus transhepatic percutaneous cholecystostomy. Hepatogastroenterology. 2010;57:12–7.

48. Van Overhagen H, Meyers H, Tilanus H, Jeekel J, Lameris J. Percutaneous cholecystectomy for patients with acute cholecystitis and an increased surgical risk. Cardiovasc Intervent Radiol. 1996;19:72–6.

49. Hatjidakis A, Karampekios S, Prassopoulos P, Xynos E, Raissaki M, Vasilakis S, et al. Maturation of the Tract After Percutaneous Cholecystostomy with Regard to the Access Route. Cardiovasc Intervent Radiol. 1998;20:36–40.

50. Vansonnenberg E, D'Agostino HB, Goodacre B, Sanchez R, Casola G. Percutaneous gallbladder puncture and cholecystostomy: results, complications, and caveats for safety. Radiology. 1992;183:167–70.

51. Garber S, Mathieson J, Cooperberg P, Macfarlane J. Percutaneous cholecystostomy: safety of the transperitoneal route. J Vasc Interv Radiol. 1994;5:295–8.

52. Mcgahan J, Lindfors K. Percutaneous cholecystostomy: an alternative to surgical cholecystostomy for acute cholecystitis? Radiology. 1989;173:481–5.

53. D'Agostino HB. vanSonnenberg E., Sanchez R., Goodacre B. Casola G. Imaging of the percutaneous cholecystostomy tract: observations and utility. Radiology. 1991;181:675–8.

54. Picus D., Burns M., Hicks M., Darcy M., Vesely T. Percutaneous management of persistently immature cholecystostomy tracts. J Vasc Interv Radiol. 1993;4:97-101; discussion 101–2.

55. Corbett C, Fyfe N, Nicholls R, Jackson B. Bile peritonitis after removal of T-tubes from the common bile duct. Br J Surg. 1986;73:641–3.

56. Saad W, Wallace M, Wojak J, Kundu S, Cardella J. Quality improvement guidelines for percutaneous transhepatic cholangiography, biliary drainage, and percutaneous cholecystostomy. J Vasc Interv Radiol. 2010;21:789–95.

Index

A

Abscess drainage
  catheter care, 47–49
  complication, 47
  contraindication, 35
  drainage technique
    Seldinger technique, 38–41
    tandem trocar drainage, 41–42
  equipment
    directional catheter, 37
    drainage catheter, 37
    fascial dilators, 37
    guidewires, 36
    needles, 36
  follow-up, 47
  imaging guidance, 37–38
  indications, 34–35
  patient preparation, 35–36
  postdrainage management, 47–49
  solid organ drainage
    hepatic abscess drainage, 44–45
    renal abscess drainage, 46–47
    splenic abscess drainage, 46
Acalculous cholecystitis, 91
Adrenal gland biopsy, 24–25
American Society of Anesthesiologists
(ASA) Physical Status Classification, 2, 3
Angioplasty balloon
  biliary strictures, 90
  gastrostomy, 75–76
Antibiotic prophylaxis, 7

B

Bile leak/biloma, 91, 96
Bile peritonitis, 91, 94, 96
Biliary dilatation, 84
Biliary intervention
  management
    benign biliary strictures, 89–90
    malignant biliary strictures, 90–91
    percutaneous cholecystostomy, 91–96
    percutaneous transhepatic cholangiography, 83–89
Biliary obstruction, 84. *See also* Transhepatic cholangiography
Biopsy. *See also* Image-guided percutaneous biopsy
  core biopsy, 18–19
  FNA, 18
Bleeding, 91
Blood urea nitrogen (BUN), 6

R.S. Arellano, *Non-Vascular Interventional Radiology of the Abdomen*, DOI 10.1007/978-1-4419-7732-8,
© Springer Science+Business Media, LLC 2011

C

Catheter dislodgement
  cholecystostomy, 96
  gastropexy, 74
Cholecystostomy
  acute calculous cholecystitis, 91
  clinical success, 91
  complication, 96
  follow-up, 94–96
  indication, 91–92
  morbidity and mortality, 91
  technique
    bladder drainage, 94
    intravenous sedation and
      local anesthesia, 92
    Seldinger technique, 93
    transperitoneal/transhepatic
      approach, 92–93
    ultrasonography, 92
Choledocholithiasis, 84
Coagulapathy, 85
Coagulation testing and factors, 5
Coagulopathy, 73
  image-guided percutaneous
    biopsy, 14
  nephrostomy, 56
  pelvis abscess drainage, 35
Coaxial technique, 19, 20, 22
Cope-locking gastrojejunostomy
  catheter, 77
Core biopsy, 18–19
Cutting needles, 15, 18–19

F

Fascial dilators
  abscess drainage, 37
  gastrostomy, 75–76
  nephrostomy, 63
  Seldinger technique, 39, 41
Fentanyl (Sublimaze), 8, 11

Fine needle aspiration (FNA), 18
Foley catheters, 72–73

G

Gastric distention, 73
Gastrojejunostomy, 77–78
Gastropexy, 74–75
Gastrostomy
  catheters, 72–73
  complications, 78
  contraindication, 72
  follow-up care, 79
  gastrojejunostomy, 77–78
  indications, 71–72
  preprocedural evaluation, 73
  technical success, 78
  technique
    angioplasty balloon, 75–76
    contrast injection, 76–77
    fascial dilators, 75–76
    fluoroscopic guidance, 74, 75
    gastric puncture, 75
    gastropexy, 74–75
    Seldinger technique, 74
    skin incision, 74
    T-fasteners, 76

H

Hemodynamic monitoring, 10
Hepatic abscess drainage, 44–45
Hydronephrosis, 60, 65. *See also*
  Nephrostomy

I

Image-guided percutaneous
  biopsy
  adrenal gland biopsy, 24–25
  complications, 19

computed tomographic
    guidance, 17
contraindications, 14
equipment
    aspiration needles, 14–15
    cutting needles, 15
indications, 13–14
liver biopsy
    focal biopsy, 20–21
    random biopsy, 19–20
magnetic resonance-guided
    biopsy, 17–18
pancreas biopsy, 23
patient preparation, 15–16
renal biopsy
    complications, 27
    nonfocal, 26
    renal mass assessment,
        25–26
    tissue analysis and thera-
        peutic option, 27
    ultrasound guidance,
        26–27
spleen biopsy
    complication, 21–22
    indication, 21, 22
    ultrasound/CT guidance, 22
technique
    core biopsy, 18–19
    fine needle aspirations, 18
ultrasound guidance, 16–17
Informed consent, 3–4, 57
Insulin, 6
International normalized ratio
    (INR), 14, 56

L
Liver biopsy
    focal, 20–21
    random, 19–20

M
Midazolam (Versed), 8
Multiplanar imaging,
    16, 18

N
Nephrolithotomy, 56, 59
Nephrostomy
    access system
        CT-guidance, 61
        fluoroscopy, 61
        ultrasound guidance,
            60–61
    anatomical consideration, 59
    complication, 67
    contraindication, 56–57
    follow-up care, 67–68
    imaging guidance, 58–59
    indication, 55–56
    patient positioning, 58
    patient preparation
        informed consent, 57
        periprocedural antibiotics,
            57
        preprocedural laboratory
            test, 57–58
    puncture site, 59
    technique
        contrast injection, 62, 63
        equipment, 61
        fascial dilators, 63
        guidewire, 62–64
        needle placement, 61–62
        nephroureteral stent,
            66–67
        nonobstructed kidney,
            64–66
        pigtail catheter, 63–64
Nephroureterostomy, 66–67
Nonobstructed kidney, 64–66

P

Pancreas biopsy, 23
Partial thromboplastin time
    (PTT), 4–5
Patient evaluation and preparation
    conscious sedation
        continuum of depth, 7–9
        fentanyl (sublimaze),
            8, 11
        midazolam (versed), 8
        physiologic measurement, 8
    postprocedure care, 10–11
    preprocedure care
        antibiotic prophylaxis, 7
        imaging studies and medical
            history, 2–3
        informed consent, 3–4
        insulin, 6
        laboratory evaluation,
            4–6
        medications, 6
        physician consultation,
            1–2
        warfarin, 6–7
    procedural care, 7–10
Pelvic abscess drainage, 42–44.
    See also Abscess
    drainage
Percutaneous abscess drainage.
    See Abscess drainage
Percutaneous biliary drainage,
    84–85. *See also*
    Transhepatic
    cholangiography
Percutaneous gastrostomy. *See*
    Gastrostomy
Percutaneous nephrostomy
    (PCN). *See* Nephrostomy
Pheochromocytoma, 25
Pneumothorax, 61
Prophylactic antibiotics, 7

R

Renal abscess drainage, 46–47
Renal biopsy
    complications, 27
    nonfocal, 26
    renal mass assessment,
        25–26
    tissue analysis and therapeutic
        option, 27
    ultrasound guidance, 26–27

S

Sedation
    conscious
        continuum of depth, 7–9
        fentanyl (sublimaze), 8, 11
        midazolam (versed), 8
        physiologic measurement, 8
    discharge criteria after, 10
Seldinger technique
    abscess drainage
        elements, 38–39
        fascial dilatation, 39, 41
        guidewire manipulation,
            39, 40
        needle choice, 39
    cholecystostomy, 93
    gastrostomy, 74
    pelvic abscess drainage, 38–41
Spleen
    abscess drainage, 46
    biopsy
        complication, 21–22
        indication, 21, 22
        ultrasound/CT guidance, 22
Subphrenic abscess, 39, 40. *See
    also* Abscess drainage
Suprapubic cystostomy
    clinical manifestation, 68
    technique, 68–69

T
Tandem trocar technique, 41–42
Tract maturation, 94–96
Transgluteal drainage, 42–44
Transhepatic cholangiography
  complications, 89
  contraindication, 85
  imaging-guided percutaneous
    access, 85
  indication, 84
  needle placement, 83–84
  percutaneous biliary drainage,
    84–85
  technique
    biliary tree opacification,
      87–88
    CHIBA needle placement,
      86–87
    external biliary drainage,
      88–89
    internal/external biliary
      drainage, 89
    intravenous conscious
      sedation/general anesthe-
      sia, 85
    patient positioning, 86
    skin incision, 86
Transvaginal aspiration, 44

U
Urinary intervention
  nephrostomy (*see*
    Nephrostomy)
  suprapubic cystostomy (*see*
    Suprapubic cystostomy)

W
Warfarin, 6–7